CW01370632

Cancer Medicine from Nature

Second Edition

*The Herbal Cancer Formulas of
Edgar Cayce & Harry Hoxsey*

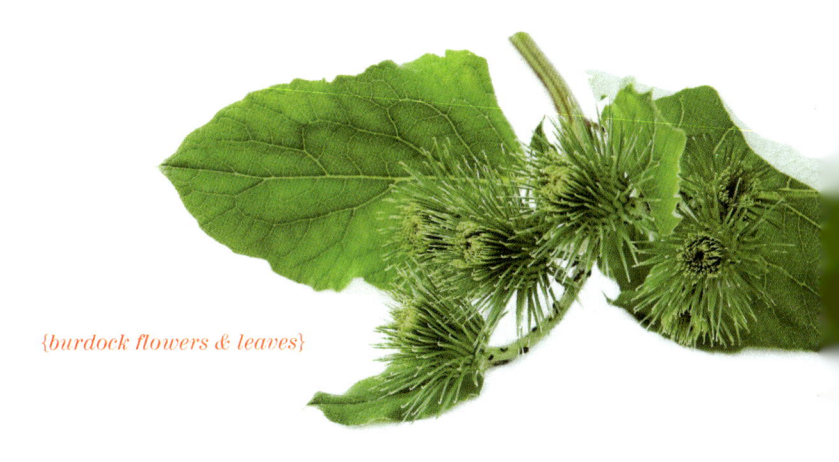

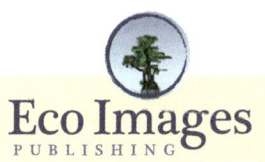

{burdock flowers & leaves}

Eco Images
PUBLISHING

by Roger Bloom

CAUTION: MANY HEALTHFUL AND EVEN LIFE-SAVING PLANTS, IF MISIDENTIFIED OR PREPARED INCORRECTLY CAN PROVE DANGEROUS. THE RESPONSIBILITY FOR PROPER IDENTIFICATION AND USE OF PLANTS MUST REMAIN WITH THE READER. PLEASE MAKE USE OF SUPERVISED CLASSES WHEN BEGINNING TO EXPLORE THIS EXCITING SUBJECT.

COPYRIGHT © 2012 BY ROGER BLOOM
SELECT PHOTOGRAPHY © 2012 BY STEVEN FOSTER
ALL RIGHTS RESERVED. NO PART OF THIS BOOK MAY BE REPRODUCED IN ANY FORM WITHOUT WRITTEN PERMISSION FROM THE PUBLISHER.

BOOK DESIGN BY TRAECY BERRYMAN
WWW.TRAECY.COM

ISBN 13: 978-1478245889
LOBRARY OF CONGRESS CATOLOG CARD NUMBER: 2012917013

PRINTED IN THE UNITED STATES OF AMERICA BY CREATESPACE
ADDITIONAL COPIES OF THIS BOOK ARE AVAILABLE FROM:
WWW.CREATESPACE.COM/3935977

PUBLISHER: ECO IMAGES, VIRGINIA BEACH, VA
WWW.ECOIMAGES-US.COM
FIRST EDITION, 2002
2ND PRINTING, 2005
3RD PRINTING, 2006
REVISED SECOND EDITION, 2012

This book is dedicated with love to

*Art & Coral Bloom
and
Gene & Joy Holmes*

*in the hope that
integrative approaches to cancer treatment
will one day be widely available to all.*

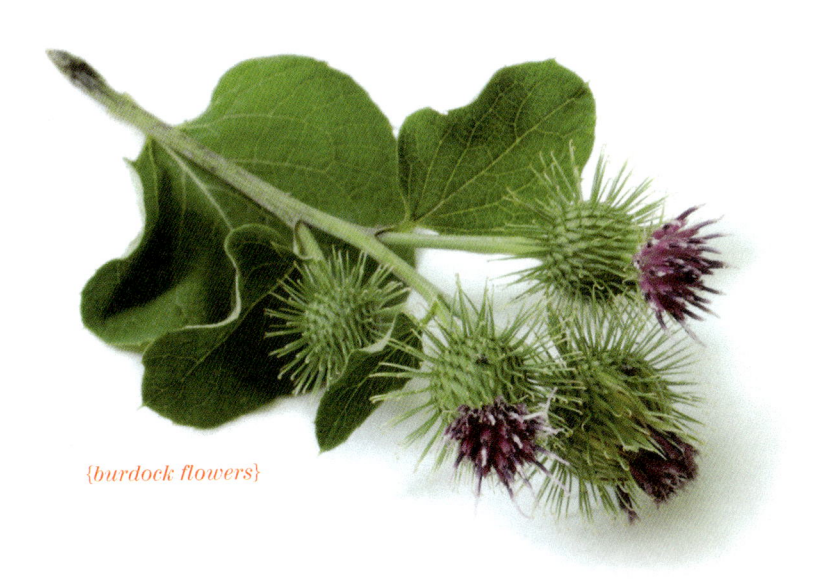

{burdock flowers}

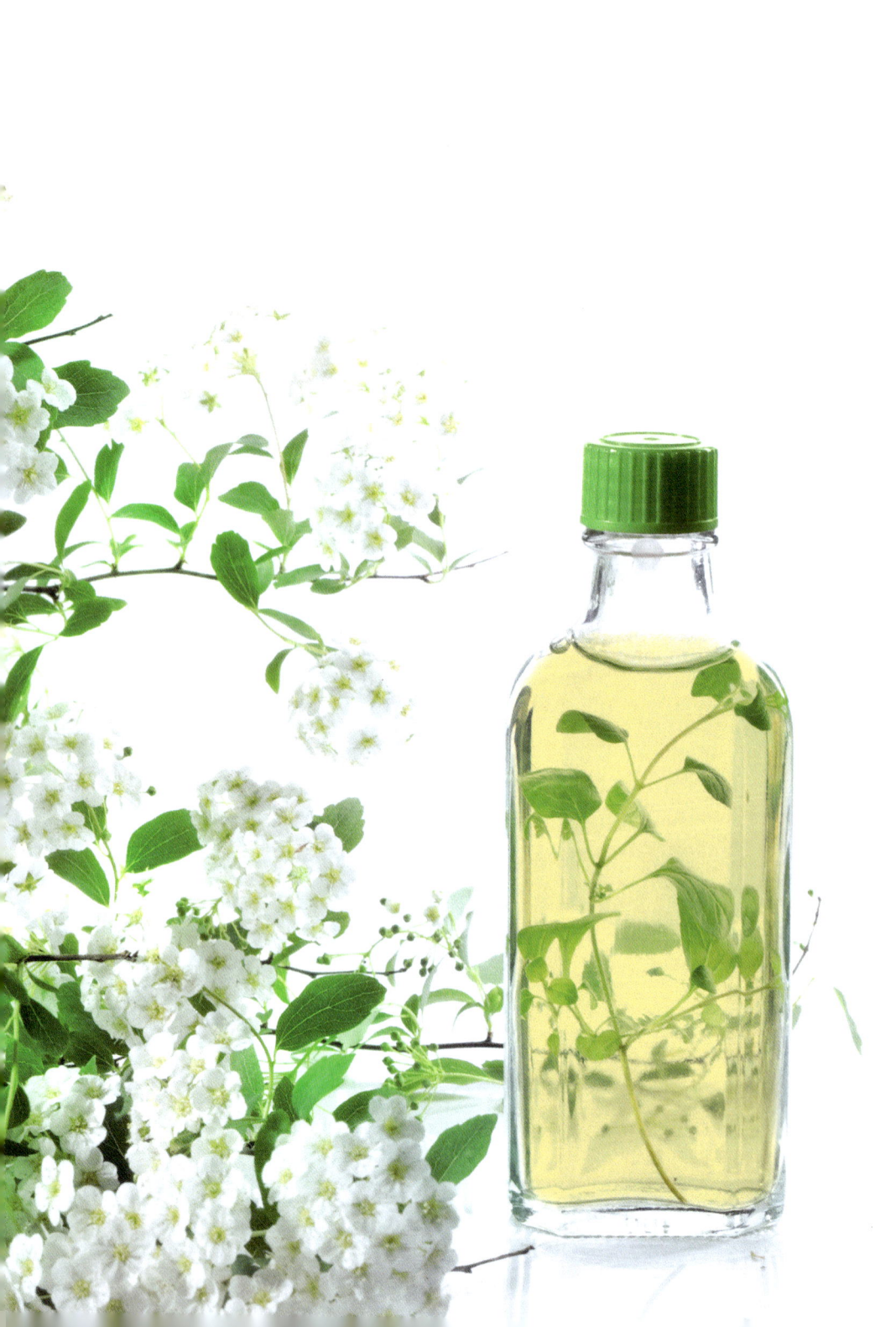

Contents

Part I } *A Legacy of Healing*

Alternatives for Those Who Seek 1
    Politics, Borders, and Healing........................... 2
    Hoxsey Therapy at the Bio-Medical Center 3
Two Pioneers in Modern Herbal Medicine
    Harry Hoxsey 4
    Edgar Cayce.. 7
Alternative Cancer Therapies 8
    Medicine from Nature 10
    The Hoxsey Formulas 10
Using Plant Medicine 14

Part II } *The Herbal Ingredients from a Modern Perspective*

Red Clover 17
Burdock 20
Poke 23
Prickly Ash 28
Stillingia 31
Buckthorn and Barberry 31
Licorice and Cascara Sagrada 33
Potassium Iodide 34
Conclusion 36

Part III } *Testimonial Correspondence*

Case One: Uterine Cancer 40
Case Two: Breast Cancer 42
Case Three: Prostate Cancer 44
Case Four: Breast Cancer, Surgery Suggested 46
Case Five: Hodgkin's Lymphoma 51
Case Six: Breast Cancer 56
Case Seven: Pancreatic Cancer 58
Case Eight: Pancreatic Cancer and Pancreatitis 61
Case Nine: Breast Cancer 63

References

Endnotes 68
Appendix A: Examples of Simple Plant Preparations 71
Resources 78
Index 83

{sassafras leaves}

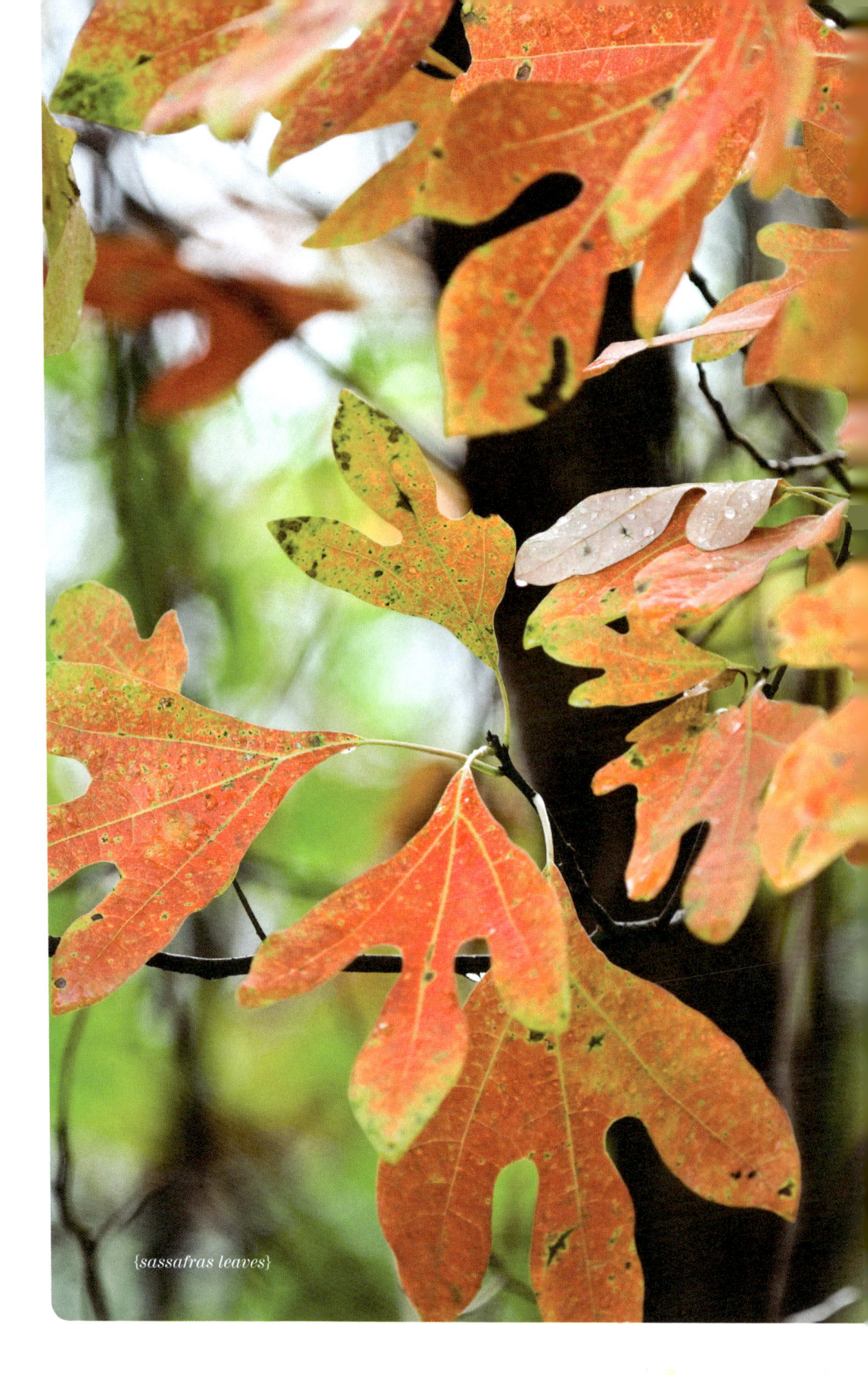

Part I } A Legacy of Healing

Alternatives for Those Who Seek

In a landmark 1971 act of congress, America declared "war" on cancer. To date, the campaign has been funded in excess of thirty billion dollars. Yet little has changed for cancer patients. Cancer today kills more than twice as many Americans each year as died in the entire Second World War. The American Cancer Society estimates over half a million Americans will die of cancer in 2012. And as these patients die, the conventional treatments available to them are often painful, poisonous, disfiguring, unsuccessful and exceedingly expensive. "Cure" rates remain controversial, yet essentially show little significant progress. Because cancer treatment as we know it in the United States has become a very big and profitable business it will be slow to change. But change it will, as evidenced by the successful grassroots political creation in the last decade of the Office of Alternative Medicine, now the National Center for Complementary and Alternative Medicine. It is, however, for those who may need options now that I wish to tell this story.

I feel a great urgency to share this information. It concerns the demonstrated promise of herbal medicines and similar alternative cancer therapies suggested in the readings of American Christian mystic, Edgar Cayce, and in the formulas of American naturopath Harry Hoxsey. I know how dearly I could have used this information some years back as my own family dealt with cancer. It seems almost daily I meet others who might benefit from such knowledge. I am saddened that this information is not more widely known. Yet I also realize the complexity of this subject. It is not only scientifically complex, but also politically charged. Any article cries out for disclaimers.

{elder berries}

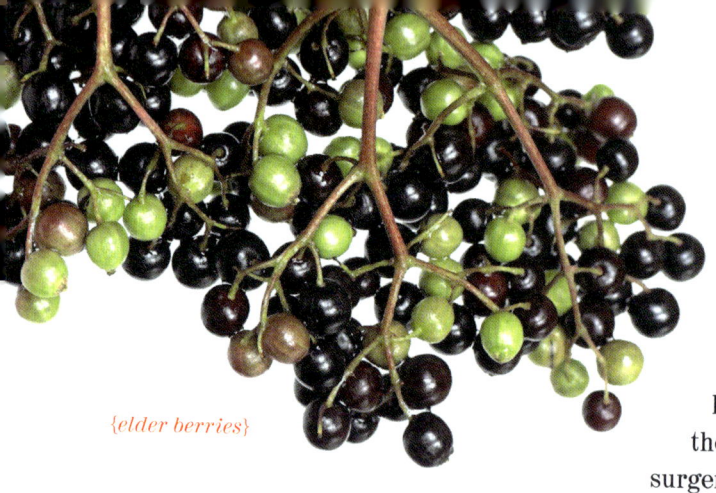

I have come to believe that eventually higher cure rates will be proven to exist for certain alternative cancer therapies, including the Hoxsey herbal therapy, than for the present standard of surgery, radiation, and chemotherapy. The information in this story, for now, remains outside the mainstream of American medicine. It has been my experience that most medical practitioners are not familiar with Edgar Cayce or Harry Hoxsey, and that fewer know of their successes or their formulas. In this story, Cayce and Hoxsey will have to bear witness to each other. The purpose of this book is to explore their herbal cancer formulas, and as importantly, to suggest the promise of nature's medicine surrounding us.

Politics, Borders, and Healing

I will begin near the end of the story, so to speak, when diverse elements began to come together in a more useful and understandable manner. In the summer of 2001, while on a business trip to San Diego, California I made an afternoon excursion across the border to Tijuana, Mexico. My purpose was to visit an alternative cancer treatment center which I had read about for years. What I witnessed on that and a subsequent visit, was the professional and compassionate application of herbal medicine against a variety of cancers. I was allowed discussion with the doctors and patients involved. I found a majority of patients claiming significant reversals of their symptoms. That experience began to tie together for me diverse streams of information and experience from a decade of personal study and my own family's illness. The plants used in the herbal formula seemed to speak to me, "*Don't you recognize us? You have read about us often in your studies. Remember the times we have healed you. Did you not believe the Native American healers? Did you not believe Edgar Cayce?*" As I absorbed the patient's stories and pondered the consequences of a successful application of plant medicine for cancer, my faith was stirred.

As I drove through Tijuana, it seemed like one of the last places a reasonable person would seek help for a serious medical problem. It's chaotic, impoverished urban sprawl is contrasted by the cleaner, more modern, more affluent San Diego within view. I had attended the University of California in San Diego, studying engineering twenty-five years earlier. I remember reading of desperate celebrities traveling to Mexican clinics to purchase laetrile and other therapies unavailable north of the border. I believed then that American medicine must certainly be more effective than anything available in Tijuana. Yet in my studies since, the evidence had led me here. Now I looked at the pretty pastel stucco colors, and the sidewalk ice cream vendors, and found it at least 'not threatening'. I couldn't escape the irony that as a citizen of the "land of the free" I had come to Mexico looking for freedom of medical information.

Hoxsey Therapy at the Bio-Medical Center

Finding the clinic was simple, and on a later visit I used public transportation from my San Diego hotel. The clinic, or Bio-Medical Center, its' proper name, is located in what was once a spacious two-story private residence on a hillside overlooking the city. I had called a few days previously to ask permission to visit and directions. Staff members had been friendly, answering all my questions in excellent English and welcoming a visit any time without an appointment. I was surprised to find that the

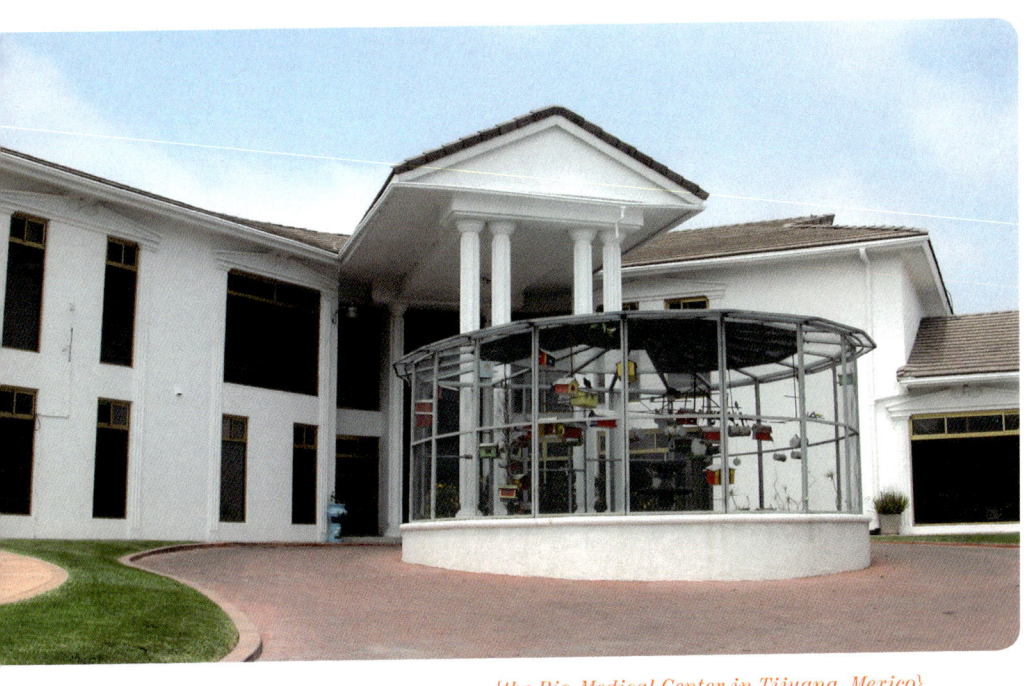

{the Bio-Medical Center in Tijuana, Mexico}

medical staff members were traditionally trained Mexican Medical Doctors. All had studied modern western medicine. They had found their way to the Bio-Medical Center through personal experience, or word of mouth. Most had been with the clinic for many years, becoming extremely experienced with cancer treatment. Because the Bio-Medical Center uses the original herbal therapies of the American Harry Hoxsey, it is often called the Hoxsey clinic.

Two Pioneers in Modern Herbal Medicine
Harry Hoxsey (1901-1974)

Born in rural Illinois, Harry Hoxsey rose from near poverty and lack of formal education to become a naturopathic physician, specializing in the treatment of cancer. His advocacy and use of controversial non-surgical and non-radiological treatments eventually involved him in a major conflict of American medical politics.

From his autobiographical account, Harry left school at the age of fifteen due to the illness of his father, a farmer and veterinary surgeon. The herbal cancer formulas with which Harry would eventually be widely associated were of veterinary origin and passed to Harry's father through the family. In the early 1900's, Harry's father had begun quietly treating patients under the supervision of local physicians. Harry was his father's closest medical assistant, and the formulas were eventually entrusted to him with the insistence that no one ever be denied treatment for financial reasons.

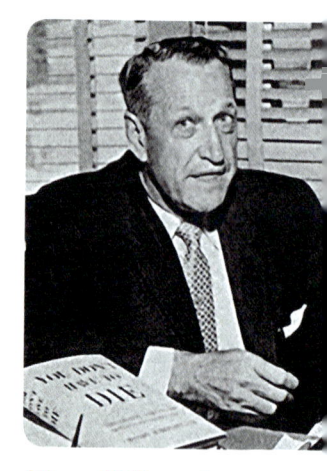

{Harry M. Hoxsey}

From the 1930's through the 1950's, Hoxsey and the doctors with whom he worked cured thousands of cancer patients, gaining widespread acclaim and publicity. In the mid 1950's, the Hoxsey clinic in Dallas, Texas was the largest private cancer clinic in the United States with more than 10,000 patients and branch clinics in seventeen states.

In order to understand Hoxsey's professional life and herbal medicines, one must consider the opposition to his methods by the medical and legal establishment of his day. A thorough treatment of this subject can be found in the book *When Healing Becomes a Crime,* and the award-winning documentary film of the same title, both written and produced by Kenny Ausabel (see the recommended reading section of this book).

Two examples of Hoxsey's battles with powerful medical interests involved the American Cancer Society and the American Medical Association. JAMA, the American Medical Association's influential journal, was edited for decades by Dr. Morris Fishbein. His writing and political activities greatly influenced national medical policy. Dr. Fishbein would later admit in court to failing anatomy in medical school, failing to complete his residency, and never having actually practiced medicine, yet he wielded enormous power through control of the journal. It provided the voice and largest revenue source of the Association. He successfully obtained his largest advertising accounts from the tobacco industry and returned their favors by promoting the health benefits of smoking. He actively worked to destroy the careers of distinguished physicians who disagreed with him. Hoxsey, who was not well educated, not a medical doctor, and often outspoken, was easily portrayed as an imposter. Dr. Fishbein, through labeling differing medical philosophies as quackery, almost eliminated the availability of chiropractic, homeopathic and eclectic medical services in the United States. He relentlessly campaigned against Hoxsey as being a dangerous fraud. Eventually, several court cases upheld Hoxsey's remedies, but did not end his harassment. Dr. Fishbein held his powerful position within the AMA from 1924 until his firing in 1950. Even after Dr. Fishbeins departure from the AMA, the organization continued to influence state medical boards to discredit alternative medical approaches, and rallied political opposition and federal agency actions against the Hoxsey clinics.

Contrary to a carefully crafted public image as a research organization, the American Cancer Society cooperated with the American Medical Association and others in discouraging new directions in cancer treatment. An example occurred in 1958, when the American Cancer Society initiated a political campaign in California to criminalize the treatment of cancer by any means other than surgery, radiation or chemotherapy. Hoxsey's second largest clinic was in Los Angeles. It was a primary target of the campaign. Following success in California, the ACS promoted similar laws across the nation. These laws made it a felony to treat cancer with alternative medicines, and remain the law of the land in most states to this day. One legacy of such actions is that current physicians know little of alternative cancer therapies, and must even discuss the subject with caution. Presently, an internet search of the Hoxsey therapy will return many false and misleading warnings prepared during this period of medical conflict, almost a half century ago.

Unfortunately for patients, as cancer treatment has become an ever larger business, medical conflicts of interest have grown. This dilemma is clearly chronicled by medical historian Dr. Ralph Moss, whose many reports, books and documentaries, include *The Cancer Industry*, published in 1989. The story of Harry Hoxsey's successful court fights with a monopolistic medical establishment during the height of McCarthyism in America is politically and personally dramatic. Evidence from the Fitzgerald special council's report to the U.S. Senate, and investigative reporter Kenny Ausabel's previously mentioned book, both do an excellent job of documenting the conspiracy of medical interests and government regulators, which thwarted several promising cancer therapies, including Hoxsey's.[1] Although successfully defended in court, Hoxsey's clinics could not operate under the constant harassment of American Medical Association controlled medical licensing boards and Federal Drug Administration interventions. Doctors who worked for Hoxsey had their licenses revoked, and medicines were restricted from transportation and the mail. The Hoxsey therapy was essentially suppressed in the United States by 1960.

Mildred Nelson, R.N., was Harry Hoxsey's head nurse at the Dallas clinic, beginning in 1946. In the early 1960's he asked her to move the clinic to Mexico and drop his name from it, in an effort to reduce controversy. Mildred became director of the Bio-Medical Center in Tijuana from its founding, in 1963, until her passing in 1999. Interestingly, she had accepted a nursing position working for Hoxsey, in Dallas, to protect her mother who was determined to give his treatment a try. Mildred thought Hoxsey was a quack and planned to expose him. Working at the clinic changed her mind and she devoted her life to the Hoxsey treatment. Mildred's mother was cured and lived into her nineties cancer free.

The medical politics of this cancer therapy, although dramatic and compelling, are not the direction of this story; rather the herbal therapy itself is. I want to consider the ingredients and formulas. And, as importantly, I want to present the reasoning by which one may come to view these herbal combinations, not as snake oil, but rather as divine gifts of sophisticated medicine.

Edgar Cayce (1877-1945)

Without hesitation I can state that the most inspiring and useful information I have come across in my life have been the records of the American Christian mystic and seer, Edgar Cayce. He provides the best documented and authenticated examples of medical clairvoyance in this century.[4] He has been called the father of holistic medicine. The thousands of medical case histories he left are computerized, indexed and easily available from a foundation, the Association for Research and Enlightenment (A.R.E.), in Virginia Beach, Virginia. Cayce's legacy convinced me of the importance of nutrition and the efficacy of herbal formulas.

Cayce did not limit himself to herbal or nutritional medicine however. From a trance-like state he accurately described his patient's complex internal conditions and provided suggestions for treatment. His recommendations often included spinal adjustment, various physical therapies, attitudinal counseling, drugs, and even surgery when indicated. He maintained that a patient's attitudes and emotions had physical manifestations which would limit or hasten recovery. His therapy was tailored to each individual. When looking at numerous patients with similar diagnoses however, parallels in treatment with minor variations can often be drawn. Over the years, as cancer reappeared in my family, I did just that.

Orthodox and alternative cancer treatment had become of keen interest to me, as both my father and mother had succumbed to the disease. My father died in the mid 1960's and my mother in the late 1990's. Both underwent surgery and radiation. My mother also had chemotherapy.

My investigation found that Cayce used many different approaches to the treatment of cancer. Among therapy modalities suggested were electrical and vibrational, oxygen (animated ash) and colored (green) light, spinal manipulation, external packs and poultices, nutritional, attitudinal, pharmacological, and very importantly, herbal.

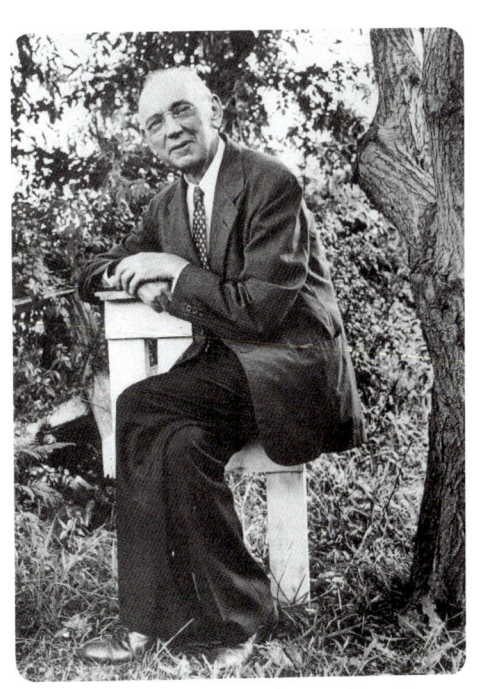

{Edgar Cayce}

At this point, because of the many therapy types and equipment required, I had difficulty focusing or helping my family use this information. My father's illness occurred while I was still a teenager, long before I was exposed to herbal medicine. My mother, living at some distance from me in her senior years, felt she had to follow her doctor's advice in a timely manner. I, unfortunately, only had generalized theories, a growing belief, and makeshift appearing alternatives to suggest. My mother's fight ended just a few years before my first visit to Mexico.

Alternative Cancer Therapies

Of course I also looked to sources other than Cayce for alternative cancer therapies and found a similar wide array of choices. These included immune therapies, nutritional therapies, metabolic therapies, and energy medicine. I discovered excellent compilations written for people trying to make treatment decisions. Favorites of mine are, *Options: The Alternative Cancer Therapy Book,* by Richard Walters[6] and *Outsmart Your Cancer,* by Tanya Pierce. Nothing is as inspiring as survivors telling their personal stories. Anthony Sattilaro M.D.'s *Recalled By Life*[7] and *The Jason Winters Story*[8] caught my attention, along with the stories of Ann Wigmore[9], Renee' Caisse[10] and others. Sattilaro, a doctor, was a terminal cancer patient that ironically found himself an impersonally treated patient in the large Philadelphia hospital where he had previously been on staff. Given up to die by his colleagues, he discovered healing in an Asian macrobiotic diet and effected a complete remission. Jason Winters, an adventurer and Hollywood stunt man, advised by his doctors that his cancer was terminal, roamed the world in search of alternatives. In combining several herbal tea mixtures, he discovered one which reversed his disease. A primary ingredient in Winters' tea was red clover blossoms. We will see them again. Ann Wigmore's memories of foraging for food amid invading armies during World War I later led her to rediscover the powerful nutritional effect of wheat grass juice. Also, Canadian nurse Renee Caisse's successful use of a native American healer's tea of burdock root began to suggest to me a hint of the grace surrounding us. Not by coincidence, the very plant ingredients used successfully by these individuals was beginning to form an herbal all-star team that I would meet again at the Bio-Medical Center.

{wild cherry fruits and leaves}

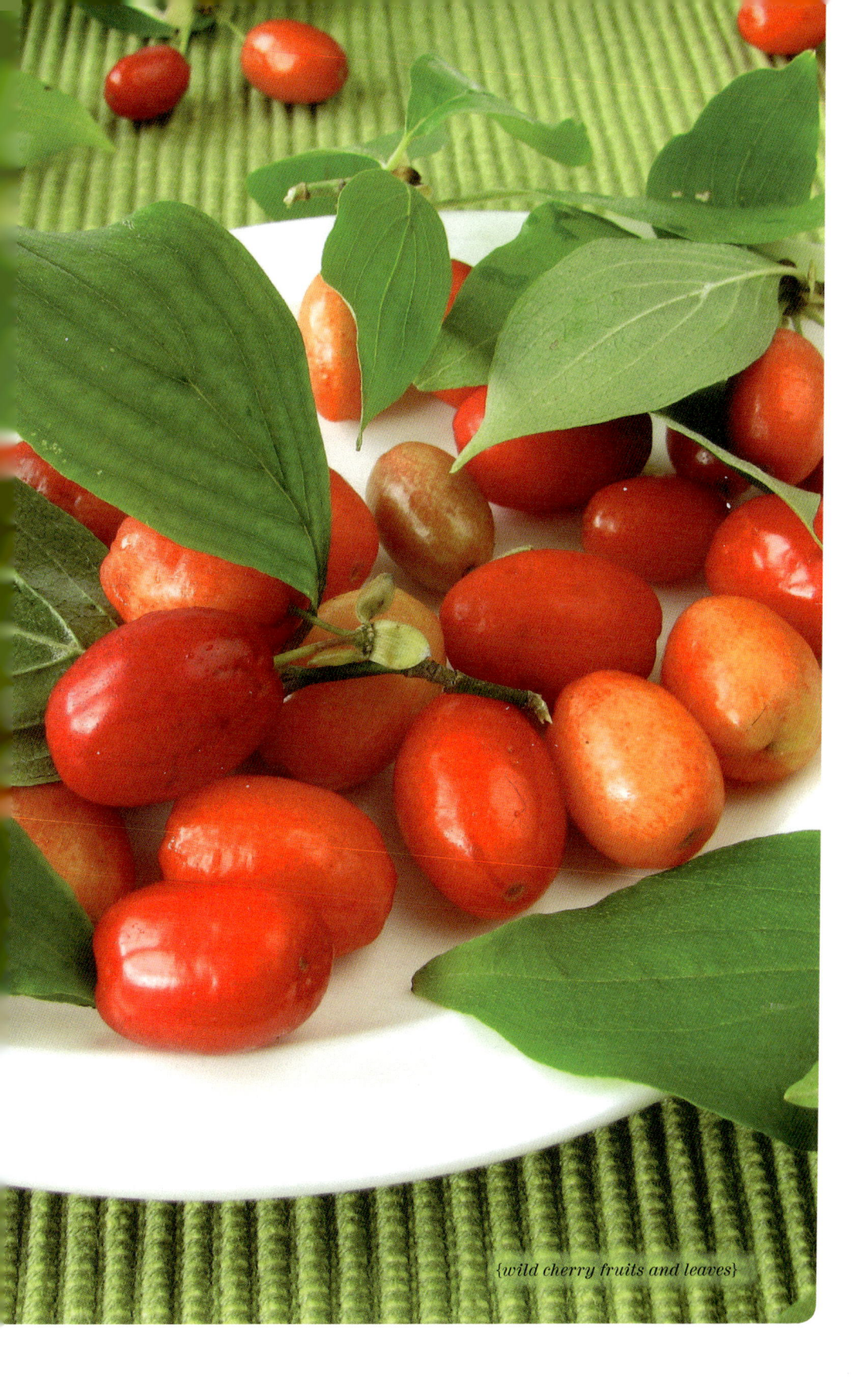

Medicine From Nature

Ten years ago I moved to an area adjacent to a state forest and a library. A growing interest in edible and medicinal plants was nurtured by walks in the forest, numerous books from the library, and enthusiastic naturalists such as Tom Brown Jr.[11], Vickie Shufer[12] and Dr. James Duke[13]. One day, passing a vacant lot where I had previously identified a number of edible and medicinal plants, I observed construction in progress for a fast food restaurant on the site. I realized then that my perspectives had been gradually changing. I knew that this isolated project was in fact only a small image of what was happening on a global scale. Instead of the prospect of food where there had previously been none, I now saw nutritious food and potential medicine being bulldozed, replaced by foods hastily manufactured for maximum profit. In many cases it having been established beyond a reasonable doubt that these very products and processes contribute to cancer and heart disease, the nation's top two killers.

I learned that it required hundreds of millions of dollars to move a drug through commercial development. Therefore, most drugs were the synthesis of one isolated ingredient manufactured in a way which was patentable and therefore profitable. The original plant from which these chemicals were isolated may have contained hundreds of synergistically useful compounds at no cost. I witnessed, on many occasions, the healing of wounds in my own family that had resisted even antibiotics using the common but powerful "weed" plantain. Later I discovered that Edgar Cayce used a plantain salve to treat external cancers. My family learned to prepare the common pokeweed, which proliferates in our yard and which will become a star later in this story, for nutritious meals. Over time I learned that many common "weeds" contained more nutrition than commercial produce at the market, and were more effective as medicine than synthesized and patented pharmaceuticals.

The Hoxsey Formulas

So what is in the herbal medicine at the Bio-Medical Center in Tijuana? It is claimed to be the exclusive home of the original Hoxsey formula. With Mildred Nelson, R.N., providing continuity of oversight from Hoxsey's original Dallas clinic, there is every reason to believe that it is. Hoxsey disclosed his formulas in court cases and in his book. We will see that current research affirms anticancer properties for its constituents, and that similar formulas have long historical use.

{buckthorn tincture}

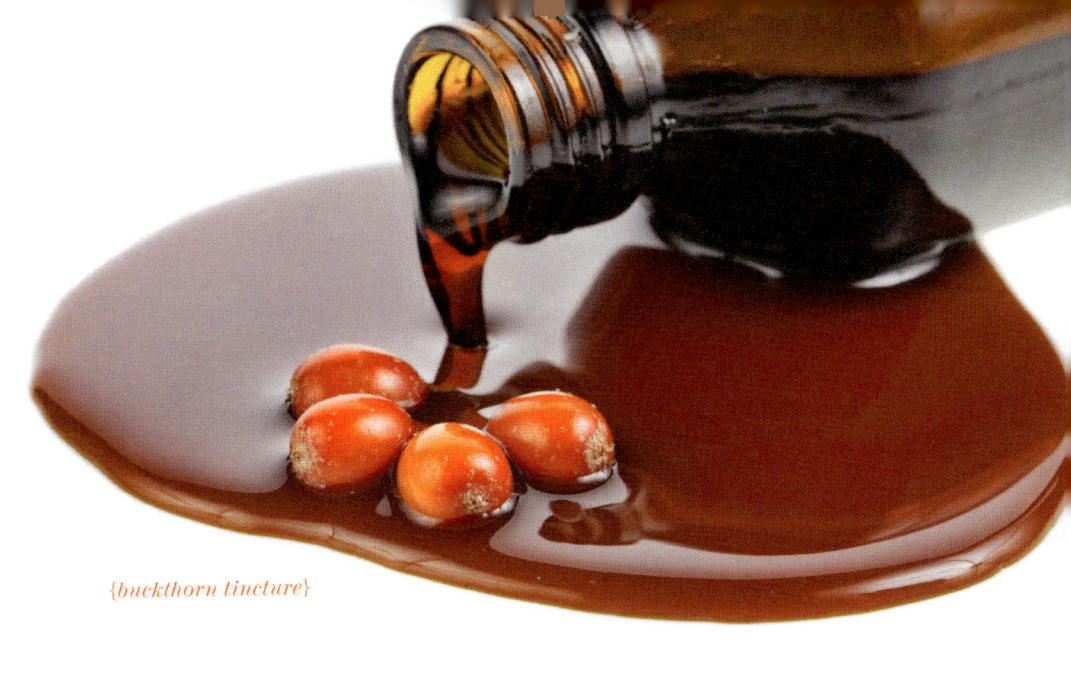

From Hoxsey's 1956 Autobiography:

"We are convinced that cancer cannot be cured successfully as an isolated phenomenon, unrelated to basic body processes. We attempt to get at the roots of the disorder, rather than deal merely with its end result. Our primary effort is to restore the body to physiological normalcy. We have a basic medicine which, taken orally, accomplishes this purpose. It stimulates the elimination of toxins which are poisoning the system, thereby corrects the abnormal blood chemistry and normalizes cell metabolism. Its ingredients are not secret. It contains potassium iodide combined with some or all of the following inorganic substances, as the individual case may demand: licorice, red clover, burdock root, stillingia root, barberries root, poke root, cascara, aromatic USP 14, prickly ash bark, buckthorn bark. It is worth noting that potassium iodide is commonly used in chronic diseases like syphilis to dissolve fibrous tissue in lesions caused by these diseases, and as preparatory action for actual treatment with arsenicals, bismuth and mercury, etc. And that the synthetic anti-coagulant Dicumarol derives from spoiled sweet clover. We prescribe the above medication in all cases of cancer, internal and external. (Except where there is evidence of latent or arrested tuberculosis, in which instance the use of potassium iodide is contraindicated.) The exact ingredients and dosage vary, depending on the individual patient's general condition, the location of the cancer and the extent of previous treatment. We have another type of medication which we apply locally in external cases. Its purpose is to halt the spread of the disease and speed the necrosis (death) of cancer cells. It is employed either as a yellow powder, a red paste or a clear solution, in accordance with the location and type of the cancer. Their formulas are not secret, either. The powder contains arsenic sulphide, yellow precipitate, sulphur and talc; the red paste has antimony trisulphide, zinc chloride and bloodroot; the liquid is trichloro-acetic acid."[14]

That Hoxsey's external formulas were effective against cancer was admitted, and never contested in the government cases against him. That Hoxsey's internal herbal formula was ineffective was the government's claim. The government, however, would not grant him an investigation. Every outside investigation which occurred supported Hoxsey's record of success. The herbal formula Hoxsey represented to the public then was as follows:

HOXSEY'S HERBAL FORMULA INGREDIENTS

licorice	stillingia
cascara sagrada	prickly ash bark
red clover	buckthorn bark
burdock	berberis root
poke root	potassium iodide

In the years since Hoxsey's depositions, a handful of additional ingredients have at times been rumored to be in the formula. Suggested additions have included chaparral, sarsaparilla, turmeric, pau d'arco, and rhubarb. While never confirmed, all would fall well within their standard herbal usages in an alterative, detoxifying formula such as Hoxsey's.

At the height of Hoxsey's business at his Dallas clinic in 1954, a group of ten physicians from around the country spent several days looking at his patients and the clinic records and made the following statement:

> "We find as a fact that our investigation has demonstrated to our satisfaction that the Hoxsey Cancer Clinic at Dallas, Texas, is successfully treating pathologically proven cases of cancer, both internal and external, without the use of surgery, radium

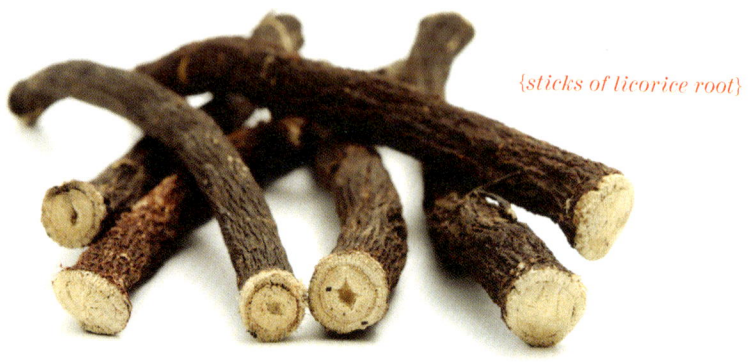

{sticks of licorice root}

or x-ray. Accepting the standard yardstick of cases that have remained symptom-free in excess of five to six years after treatment, established by medical authorities, we have seen sufficient cases to warrant such a conclusion. Some of those presented before us have been free of symptoms as long as twenty-four years, and the physical evidence indicates that they are all enjoying exceptional health at this time.

We as a Committee feel that the Hoxsey treatment is superior to such conventional methods of treatment as x-ray, radium, and surgery. We are willing to assist this Clinic in any way possible in bringing this treatment to the American public. We are willing to use it in our office, in our practice on our own patients when, at our discretion, it is deemed necessary.

The above statement represents the unanimous findings of this Committee. In testimony thereof we hereby attach our signatures.

S. Edgar Bond, M.D.
Richmond, IN

Willard G. Palmer, M.D.
Seattle, WA

Hans Kalm, M.D.
Aiken, SC

A.C.Timbs, M.D.
Knoxville, TN

Frederick H. Thurston, M.D., D.O.
Boise, ID

E.E.Loffler, M.D.
Spokane, WA

H.B.Mueller, M.D.
Cleveland, OH

R.C.Bowie, M.D.
Fort Morgan, CO

Benjamin F. Bowers, M.D.
Ebensburg, PA

Roy O.Yeats, M.D.
Hardin, MT"[15]

Let us return now to the Bio-Medical Center. When I arrived I was greeted, shown around and invited to talk to any patients who wished and to the staff. Being an out-patient facility, most visitors arrive early to accomplish as much as possible before returning across the border for the night. In the morning, exams are given, x-rays and blood work are done, and there is a friendly small cafe to have breakfast or lunch. Patients were very willing to tell their tales. Many told me of cancers cured years previously; they return now only for check-ups. In the afternoon doctors meet individually with patients—and follow up with treatment.

There was a business office where I inquired about the cost of treatment. Basically all diagnosis, treatment, and an initial six months or so worth of medicine is approximately $1,000. Lifetime maximum expense is capped at approximately $3,500. It is the policy of the clinic that no one is refused treatment because of financial problems.

I was surprised at the worldwide clientele of the clinic and at how people in the United States had learned of it through word of mouth. I had some questions about the herbal formula for the doctors. I, of course, already knew the publicly stated plant ingredients. I also knew that Hoxsey claimed to modify slightly his formula at times. I brought up the question of exactly how the tonic was formulated. Of course I knew this was proprietary, but I was secretly afraid someday the clinic would close and the recipe would be lost. Was it an alcoholic tincture or made like a tea? I did not get a definitive answer. But the doctor suggested that if I used standard herbal methods I would probably be very close. He also stressed that alcohol was not in the formula, and, if taken while on the formula, would negate it. Typical dosage was a teaspoonful four times daily, before meals and at bedtime. However, the dosage was modified by experience, depending on the location and stage of the cancer.

An alcoholic or glycerin tincture is the standard method of making herbal formulas. The alcohol draws the plant properties out and holds them in suspension without refrigeration until needed. When mixed with another liquid for patient consumption, the alcoholic content is minute.

I looked again at the Edgar Cayce readings. Many times he prescribed formulations of herbs as alcoholic tinctures. Yet, as often, he provided directions to prepare infusions, that is to simmer but not boil the ingredients in water producing a fluid extract. And often to this water based concentrated "soup" Cayce added a few ounces of alcohol with balsam of tolu or balm of gilead as a preservative and digestive aid.

Using Plant Medicine

In the next section we will examine the ingredients within the Hoxsey and Cayce herbal formulas. Similarities in these formulations will be highlighted, as will supportive historical records, and recent scientific research. The question may arise: *given the individualized nature of Cayce's use of plant medicine, and the unavailability of early American medical formulas, is it really possible for an average person to make practical use of this information?* The answer is a definite yes.

In the case of an actual or suspected diagnosis of cancer, the purpose of this book is to provide perspective, information and resources to individuals and their physicians. My personal experience of the Hoxsey protocols is extremely favorable. I believe that their value derives from over seventy years' experience, specialized medical staff (cognizant that they are trained and licensed in a foreign country), affordable costs, and their ability to act synergistically with concurrent therapies.

What about the more desperate situation of someone too poor, or too sick, or simply too far from this help? Here I see the great mercy and promise of plant medicine. The nutrition and medicine is in fact all around us. It is all around the world as well. European, Asian, and African traditions have similar plants available. In my experience, an average citizen with this priceless knowledge often receives care superior in many respects to that available to the very rich and powerful. The testimonials within this book describe such experiences. The sophistication of nature is not yet exceeded in human practice. As the greatest of all healers reminded men of his age, *"Consider the lilies of the field…. Surely Solomon in all of his glory was not arrayed as one of these!"*

My own family has often followed the methods suggested in the Edgar Cayce readings for preparing medicinal plants (Examples included in this book include Readings 4138-1 in the section on red clover, and 5521-1 in the section on poke). These same plants make excellent teas, as described in popular herbal texts, such as Jethro Kloss' *Back to Eden*. Health food stores and the internet market herbs as both medicinal teas and in liquid tincture and homeopathic forms. Simpler yet, many of these plants are edible as cooked or raw vegetables. Widely available texts, such as the Peterson Field Guides, can help with plant identification and safety. The ingredients for more complex herbal formulas can be procured in dried form from reputable herbalists online. Suggested websites are listed in the Resources section at the back of this book.

Let us get started then looking more closely into what history and science reveal concerning the healing properties of these very special plants.

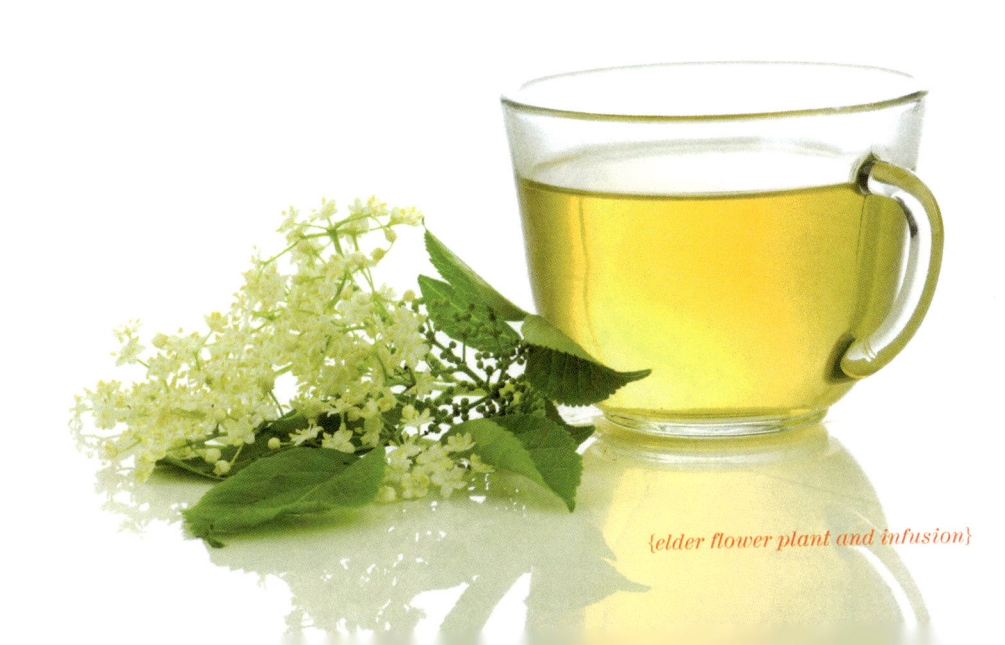

{elder flower plant and infusion}

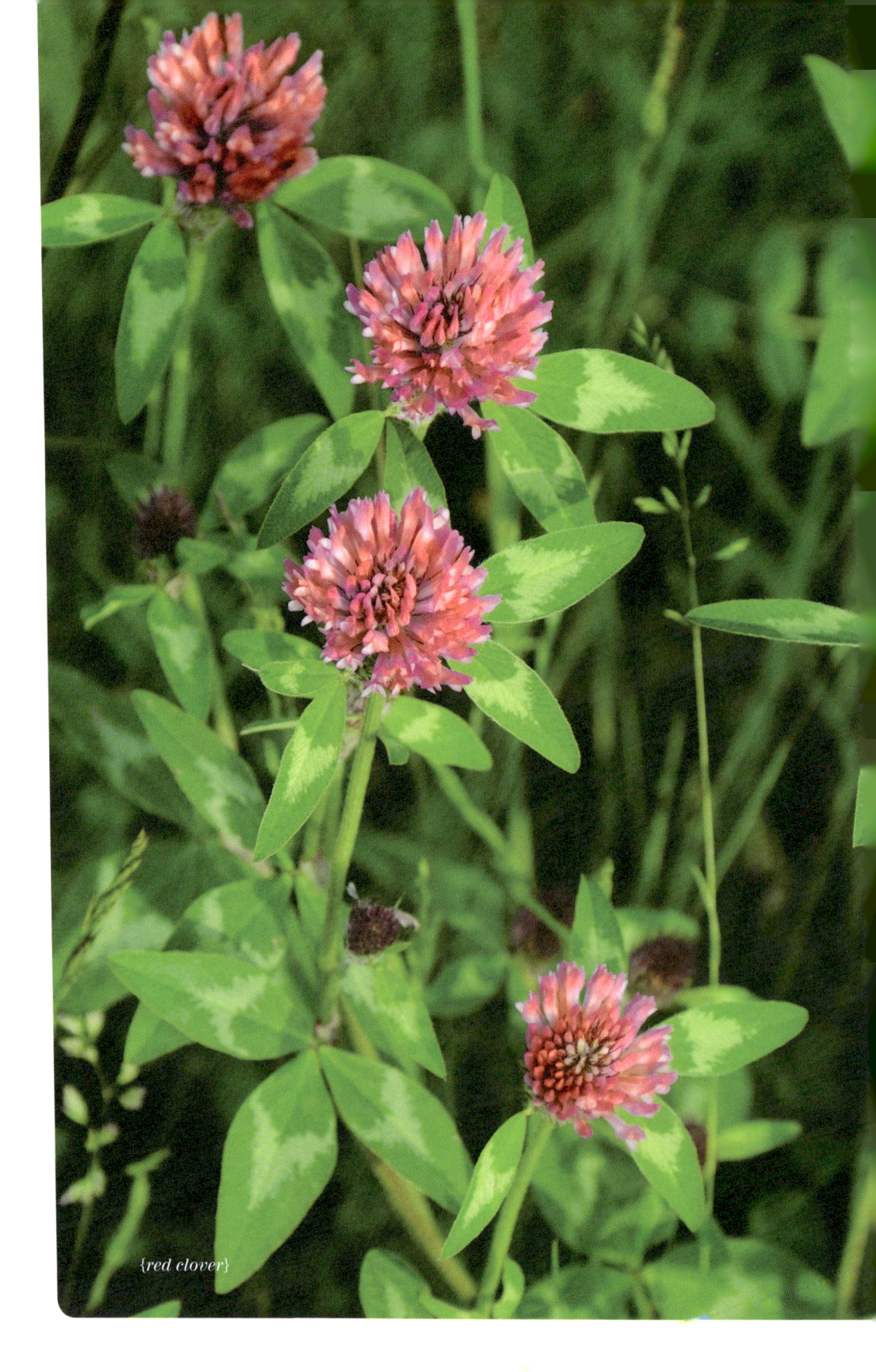

{red clover}

Part II } Herbal Ingredients From a Modern Perspective

Red Clover {*Trifolium pratense*}

Red clover has a long history as a blood purifier in herbal medicinal formulas. The National Cancer Institute's Jonathan Hartwell reported that thirty-three cultures around the world use red clover to treat cancer.[16] NCI research has found at least four anti-tumor components in red clover, including the currently medically popular phytoestrogen genistein. Testing of 150 herbs for phytoestrogen activity, published in 1998, found two Hoxsey herbs, red clover and licorice, along with soy within the six most active. Consumption of the same isoflavones in soy is currently suspected of reducing the incidence of leukemia and cancers of the breast, lung and prostate. It would also suggest that red clover could be expected to act to restrict tumor growth anti-angiogenically, similar to the popular but toxic drug Tamoxifen[17].

The famous American herbalist, Jethro Kloss (1863-1946), in his book *Back to Eden,* considered red clover "one of God's greatest blessings to man; very pleasant to take and a wonderful blood purifier … an exceedingly good remedy for cancer on any part of the body."[18] Kloss includes several successful case histories. His use of red clover alone as a tea for cancer is reminiscent of the account of Jason Winters. Interestingly, Kloss, in cases of cancer, also combined red clover with two other Hoxsey herbs, burdock and poke, as well as yellow dock.

Herbal medicine reached its greatest acceptance in America at about the turn of the last century with the eclectic practitioners. Eclectic physicians were equals in training with other physicians of the period. Francis Brinker, a naturopathic scholar investigating the Hoxsey formula, found evidence that except for the ingredients buckthorn and licorice, the

Hoxsey formula was identical to an earlier red clover based eclectic formula published in 1890 by Parke, Davis and Co. called a Syrup Trifolium Compound (*Trifolium pratense* being the botanical name for red clover)[19].

Here are two examples of Cayce readings from the 1920's, which suggest herbal formulas very similar to Hoxsey's. In the first case the patient had a condition which had thinned the walls of the small intestine, allowing toxins to reenter the body. Note the use of the Hoxsey herbs stillingia, poke and red clover in combination. For those not used to the Cayce readings, the difficult syntax is the result of a literal dictation having been taken while Cayce spoke from a sleep-like state.

FROM CAYCE READING 4387-1

Then, to bring the normal forces to this body, it would be necessary to take in the system those properties which will give the expectancy of the equalized circulation, equalized nerve distribution, equalized forces, and give the body in its functioning, especially in the region of the peyer's gland that necessary to so thicken the walls as prevent this leakage, or this toxin from disturbing the body. Then, we would take this—to four ounces of peptotone, or simple syrup, add:

fluid extract yellow dock root	½ ounce
fluid extract stillingia	½ ounce
fluid extract poke root	1/4 ounce
fluid extract red clover	½ ounce
oil of sassafras	5 minims
essence of tolu	20 minims

Shake the solution well together before each dose is taken. The dose would be half a teaspoonful in water, or direct, twice each day, mornings on arising, evenings before retiring.[20]

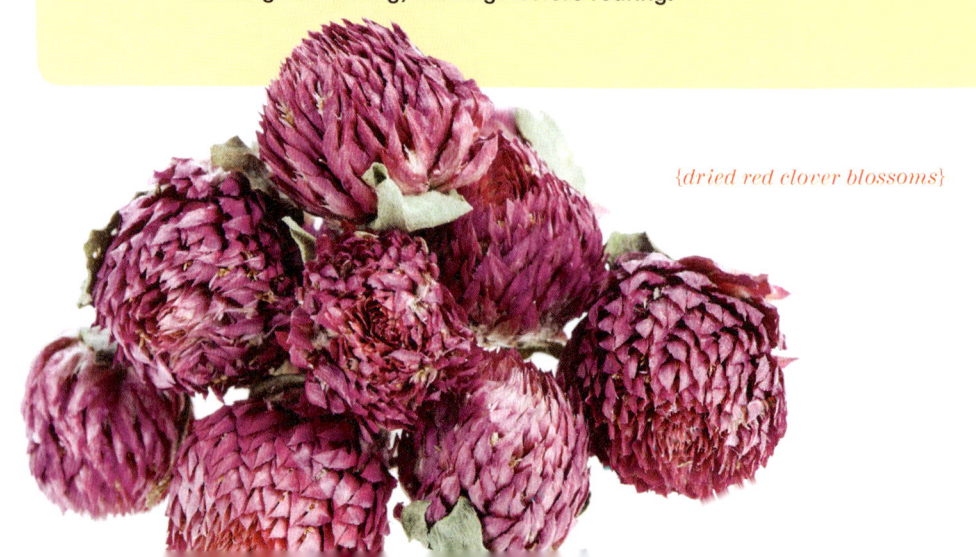

{dried red clover blossoms}

In the following reading for a woman suffering from nerve damage following pelvic surgery, as well as difficult kidney function, and inflammation of the liver, a similar formula was suggested. Note again, the additional Hoxsey herbs burdock root and prickly ash bark, along with the red clover.

FROM CAYCE READING 4138-1

First, prepare the system that corrections may be made with incentives created in system for normal functioning of organs. Then take this: To one gallon of rainwater, add:

wild cherry bark (fresh bark)	2 ounces
yellow dock root	1 ounce
burdock root	1 ounce
green, red, or sweet clover blossom	1 ounce
prickly ash bark, green preferred	1 ounce
mandrake root	20 grains
buchu leaves	30 grains
elder flower	4 ounces

Reduce by simmering (not boiling) to one quart. Strain while warm and add 4 ounces grain alcohol, with 3 drams of balsam of tolu cut in it, with 2 drams of balm of gilead. Shake solution well before taking each dose, which should be two teaspoonfuls four times each day, before meals, before retiring. Eat no meats, save fowl or fish. As much vegetable matter as is consistent for the body. Whole wheat or those properties easily digested in system. After these properties have been taken in system, and the whole quantity taken, use the vibration that would be accorded the system by the deep manipulation through osteopathic forces, with local treatment with the violet ray electrode. Do that. We will bring the normal conditions to this body."[21]

It is noteworthy that Cayce most often combined red clover with prickly ash bark, another of the Hoxsey herbs, as well as with yellow dock root, one of the most widely used herbs for blood purification.[22] Cayce consistently stressed the importance of nutritional caution while detoxifying the body. A primary goal of herbal cancer treatment is the enhancement of nutrient assimilation and toxin elimination. The Bio-Medical Center also provides dietary guidelines that include the complete avoidance of pork, vinegar, refined sugar, tomatoes, carbonated drinks and alcohol during treatment.[23]

Burdock {*Arctium lappa*}

Burdock root was a primary ingredient in Canadian nurse Renee Caisses' successful anticancer tea, based on an Ojibwa Indian recipe.[24] The famous herbalist, Eli Jones, mentioned burdock for treating cancer in his publications early in the twentieth century. Patricia Spain Ward's report for the Congressional Office of Technology Assessment (OTA) in the late 1980's mentions significant and successful anti-tumor research findings involving burdock in both Hungary and Japan.[25] Research botanist, James Duke, who during his career at USDA extensively studied plant medicine, has suggested that two lignans in burdock, arctigenin and trachelogenin, may be important reasons for burdock being useful in the treatment of leukemia and lymphoma. He also notes that among quantities of polysacharides with immune modulating activity in burdock is the prebiotic inulin, which promotes digestive system health.[26]

Cayce suggested burdock in approximately 160 readings.[27] The following reading for a patient with throat cancer included four Hoxsey ingredients: burdock, stillingia, poke and potassium iodide. This reading included an intriguing prescription for energy medicine and a complex but descriptive survey of the source and spread of the patients' cancer, beginning in the throat where cellular forces had surrounded an irritated region that later became malignant.

FROM CAYCE READING 4695-1

In the blood supply, we find this deficient in the rebuilding properties and an excess of the white blood supply, with a deficiency in the red blood, and that bacilli carried in the blood stream showing the cause, the character, of conditions as exist in the system, for the system attempts to create that necessary to war against the ravages of the sarcoma germs in the blood supply ... this produces the condition in blood supply, the condition over the whole system, and especially that as causes the condition in the circulation through the capillary ... the specific condition as found in the cuticle, for with the system attempting to eliminate, and so much of the leukocyte forces used in the destruction of the bacilli in blood supply, the capillary circulation becomes clogged and choked, and dross left without the elimination being properly cared for. *In the nerve system,* we find in this much of the condition of taxation, for with the vital forces in body being attacked by these bacilli, the nerve centers become depleted in their

reading continued on next page

{burdock}

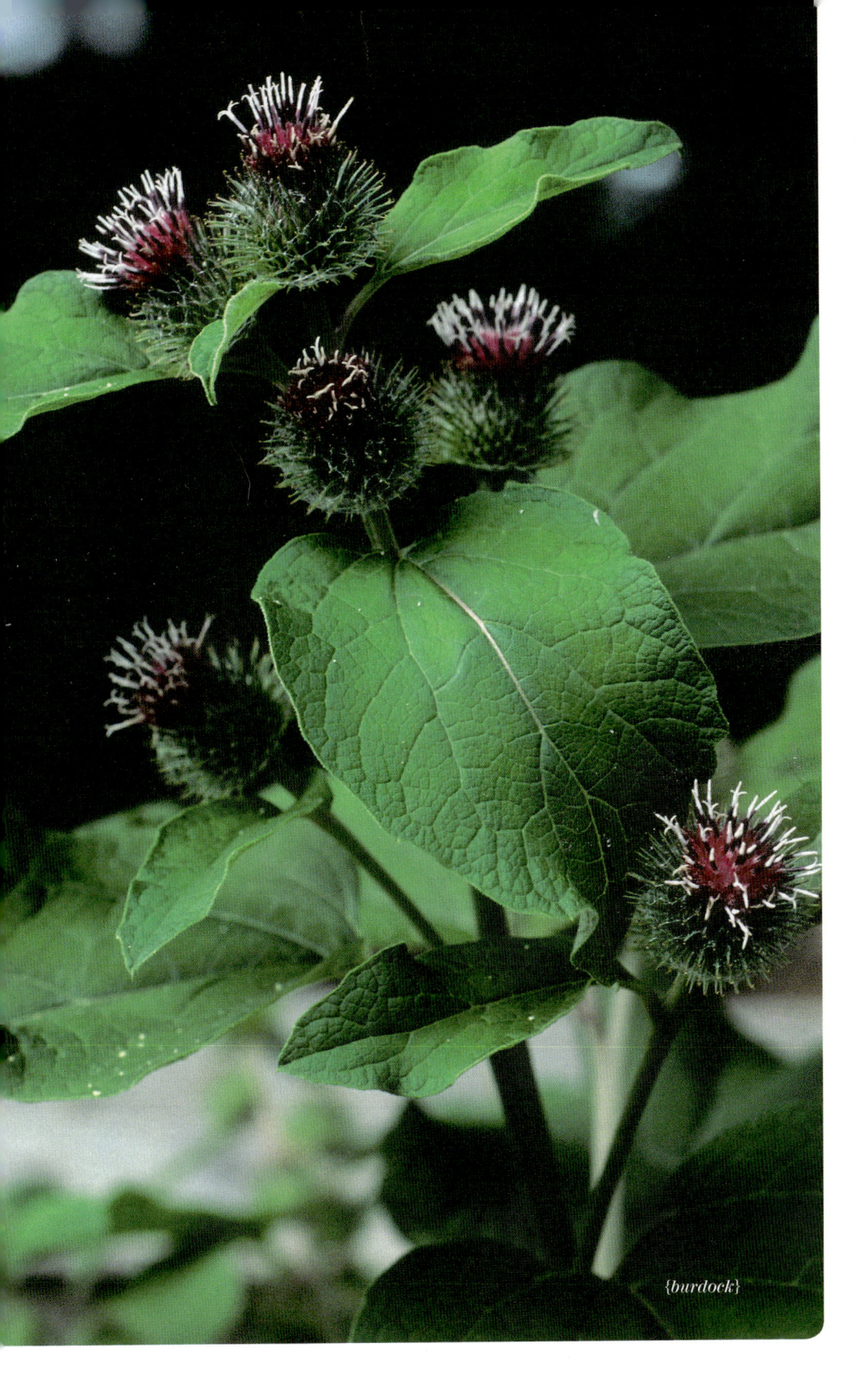

Cayce Reading 4695-1, continued from previous page

ability to function in the normal manner. Hence the tired debilitation at times that appears in the body, the feelings as if there is no use to fight against existing condition, lack of vital forces in nerve supply to meet the needs of the physical forces in the body. *In the organs of the body,* in the throat lungs and larynx: In the portion of the throat at the base, or root, of tongue, we find this condition where cellular forces show the surrounding of those conditions producing the ravages in the system, first produced by too much of certain elements in the system as taken for cathartics, and with other stimulation produced the irritation that brought about the condition which separates itself, and became the germ forces as created in the system itself ... In the functioning of other organs, we find those of the system that produce the change in circulation by the action of that organ's secretions, as we find in spleen, pancreas, liver and kidneys. All engorged to meet the needs of the system, a normal condition for existing conditions in the body. These conditions may be assisted and the condition brought to that of little effect in system if cared for in proper manner. Then do this—we would take first in the system these properties:

tincture wild cherry bark	½ ounce
tincture stillingia	½ ounce
tincture yellow dock root	½ ounce
tincture of poke root	½ ounce
tincture of burdock root	½ ounce
iodide potassium	¾ ounce
sufficient simple syrup to make	6 ounces

Shake solution well together until all is dissolved. The dose would be half a teaspoonful four times each day—letting one dose be just before retiring. And apply to the body through the solar plexus center, and at the second cervical, the plates or vibrations that will be found in the Abrahams Osculator (Abrams' Oscillator) for sarcoma germ. This will, within three to five weeks, reduce the condition to that of almost nil. Then the general health afterwards must be kept. We will find through these forces we will bring the betters conditions for this body."[28]

Recent clinical research in energy medicine is validating therapies similar to those advocated by Dr. Albert Abrams and Edgar Cayce (See *frequency specific microcurrent* in the Internet Resources section of this book, page 78).

Poke {*Phytolacca americana*}

In a 1998 research paper, the official journal of the American Society of Microbiology reported that an extremely promising anti-viral protein had been derived from poke, which has so far proven more than 100 times more effective against the HIV virus than any previous substance.[29] Poke is the common rural potherb eaten by foragers, as immortalized in the country rock classic "Poke Salad Annie." Perhaps God is again glimpsed here providing effective medicine from nature. My family has dined on the pokeweed from our backyard for years. However, it is very important to understand that if not prepared properly, poke can be harmful. Parts of the plant contain strong alkaloid poisons.

Here are the rules. Pick young green shoots and leaves in the spring from very small plants (less than 9" tall) and boil in water (I do it twice), throwing away the water. Here is how Edgar Cayce described it for a patient with cancer:

FROM CAYCE READING 3515-1

> Eat very young poke—the tender shoots of the pokeweed to act as a purifier for the body. Prepare it in this manner: When cutting sufficient to make a small dish or salad, put in cold water and let come to a boil. Strain or drain off, as in a colander—or put in a colander and let all the juice drain off. Then prepare or cook the remaining leaves with other greens, especially such as lamb's tongue and wild mustard-about an equal quantity. This eaten once a week will purify the whole body.[30]

FROM CAYCE READING 3331-1

> ... include all forms of leafy green—as poke—as this is very tender, but be careful how it is prepared. Put the tender poke leaves in plain water and allow to come almost to a boil, pour off the water or drain and then the leaves can be mixed with any other greens. The activity of these would be purifying, in such a way that will be found in few other such greens or vegetables.[31]

Poke was considered the most useful herbal medicine for various cancers by the famous eclectic physician, Eli Jones.[32] Jones was an 1870 graduate of the Eclectic Medical College of Pennsylvania and an 1871 graduate of Dartmouth Medical School. In 1911 Jones authored *Cancer, Its Causes, Symptoms and Treatment,* subtitled, "The Results of Over Forty Years' Experience in the Medical Treatment of this Disease."[33] Jones' text,

{poke berries}

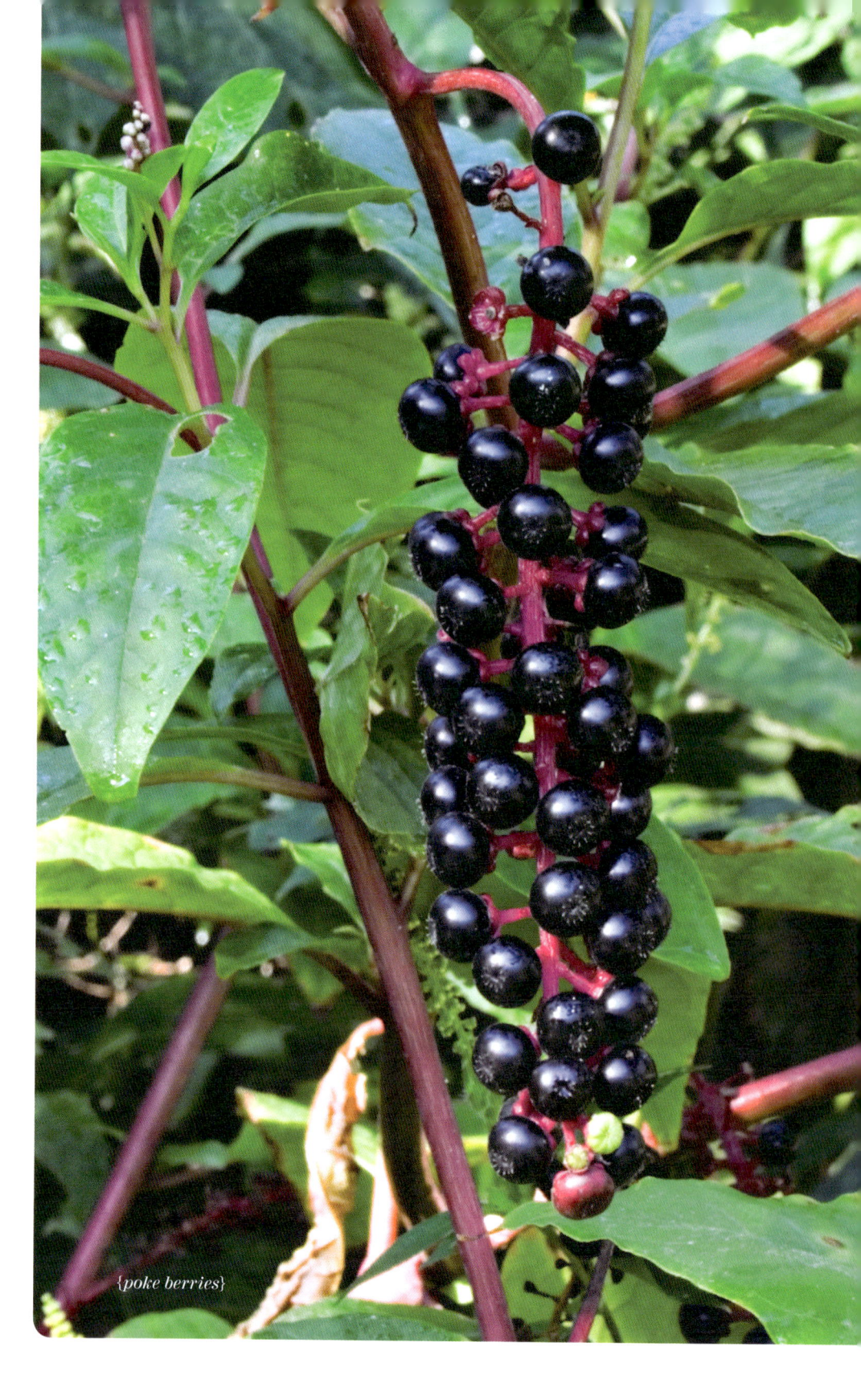

including plant-based formulas, is considered a foundation of modern oncology abroad, yet is studied little in the United States. Jones did not believe that one formula fit all cancers. Science writer Ralph Moss, in his 1998 book *Herbs Against Cancer,* notes Jones' positive experience with poke in cases of lymphoma and cancers of the breast, throat, and uterus.[34]

Poke was used by the Penobscot Indians of Maine and the Rappahannock Indians of Virginia against cancer.[35] When Patricia Spain Ward researched the Hoxsey herbs for the Office of Technology Assessment, she found twenty-one articles in respected journals, including *Lancet, Pediatrics* and *Nature,* describing the mitogenic activity of pokeweed as an immune system trigger.[36]

Cayce specified poke in approximately fifty cases.[37] Noteworthy is that among companion ingredients most often used with poke were the Hoxsey herbs stillingia, burdock, and potassium iodide.

The following treatment was suggested for an individual with swollen legs, feet covered with running skin sores, and diagnosed as having cancer. Interestingly, Cayce found the condition not actually cancerous but a case of serious systemic nightshade and mercury poisoning.

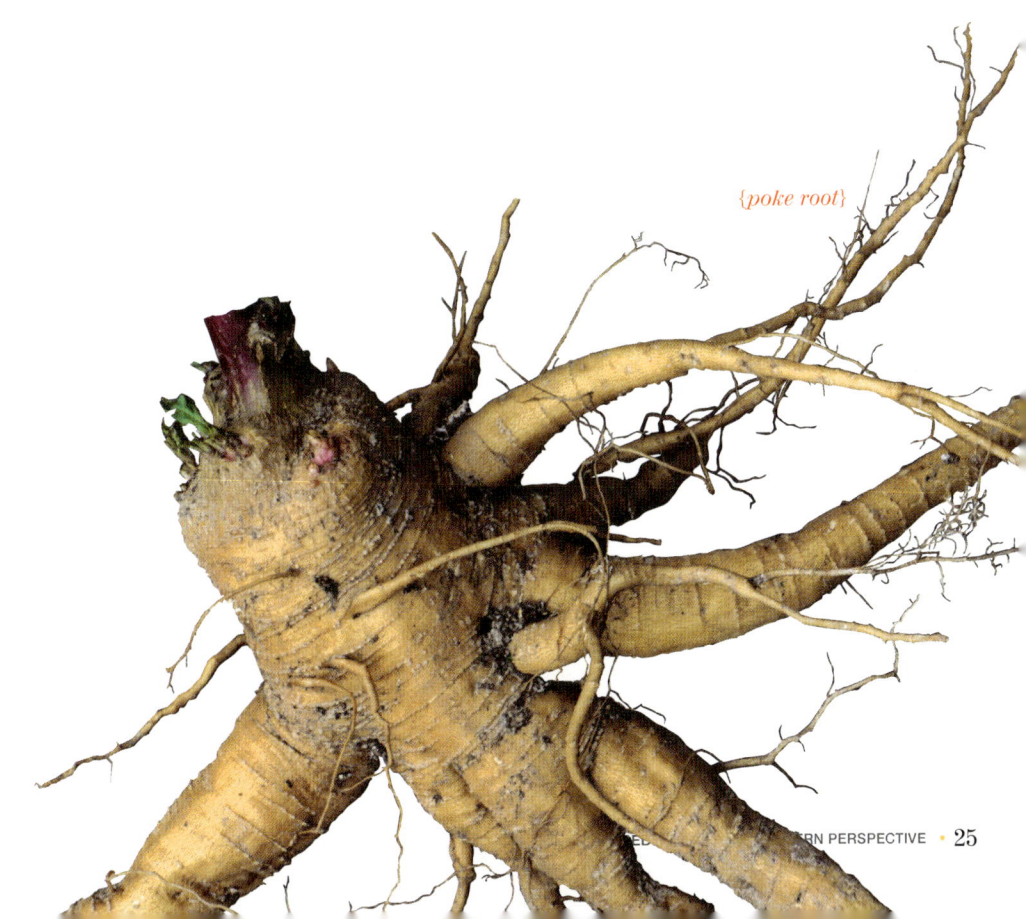

{poke root}

FROM CAYCE READING 5521-1

> ... in the lower extremities that of an aggravated ... condition that is so set in system that the condition itself reproduces itself in the form of bacilli as is shown ... Not that of the particular condition as would be termed cancerous condition, yet in this malignant form and way we find this shows something of that nature, without the wasting condition as is usually produced ... This is not the sarcoma germ. Rather that which would be produced from a dew poison, or nightshade poison, or from as we find that which produced this in the system is from taking mercury and nightshade in the system at the same time, and it produces a poison in the extremities and turned aside, as it were, the elimination in the capillary circulation, and the lymphatic glands becoming involved and poisoned. All this combined produces this condition. This in the malignant state is the accentuated, aggravated, condition in both the blood supply, in the capillaries of the extremities and in the lymphatic circulation. Hence the pus and the inflammation. Now we find this condition may be assisted, and, if properly handled and taken, may be eliminated entirely in and from the system. This will, of necessity, include all form of perfect elimination being set in the system, especially that in the emunctory circulation in liver and in kidneys, without producing in the organs themselves the incentive to accentuate the condition in the functioning organs ...

Cayce then gave instructions for an external paste of plantain leaves and oil to be alternated with the juice of the common milkweed plant and applied to the edges of the patient's external sores. For the internal conditions he prescribed the following:

> ... then to one gallon of rainwater, add:
>
> | | |
> |---|---|
> | sarsaparilla | 4 ounces |
> | wild cherry bark | 2 ounces |
> | calisaya bark | 2 ounces |
> | mandrake root | 30 grains |
> | buchu leaves | 20 grains |
> | elder flower | 2 ounces |
> | poke root | 10 grains |
>
> Reduce by simmering (not boiling) to one quart. Strain while warm and add four ounces of grain alcohol, with two drams of balsam of tolu cut in it ...

Cayce added hygiene and dietary instructions.

> ...Do this. We will bring the body to the better condition and eventually eliminate these poisons entirely from the system.[38]

Of course, we do not always have follow up information on the Cayce patients. But many wrote Cayce back to say that they had been helped. Personal patient testimonies from Hoxsey's history are voluminous.[39] The "simple plant" formulas suggested by Cayce, Hoxsey and others have proven to be powerful and not simple at all. In probably the largest listing of such plants and their uses, the National Cancer Institute's Jonathan Hartwell, in his *Plants Used Against Cancer*, lists every

{poke flowers}

one of the Hoxsey herbs with multiple citations.[40] James Duke, a USDA botanist, in reviewing the Hoxsey formula noted that all of the herbs showed anti-microbial activity, and eight had demonstrated anti-tumor activity in controlled laboratory animal tests.[41]

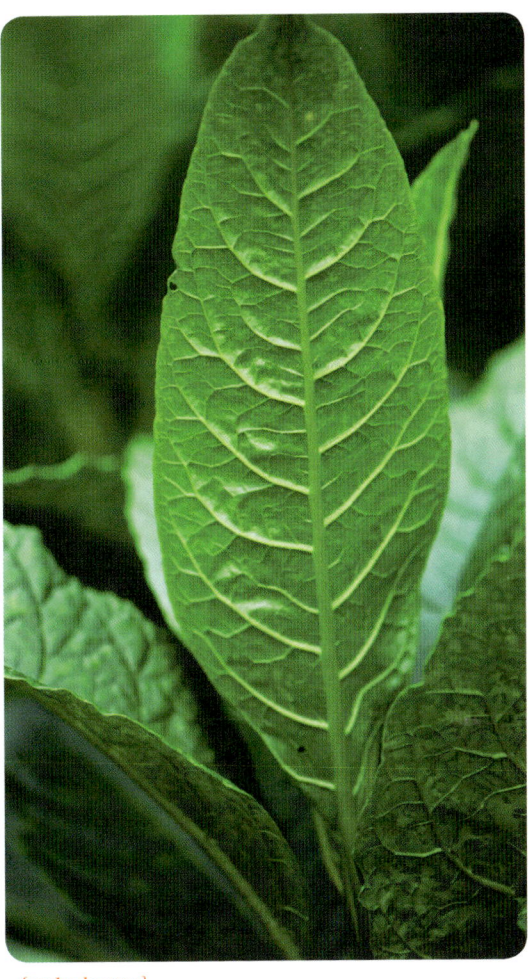

{poke leaves}

Prickly Ash {*Zanthoxylum americanum*}

James Duke notes that prickly ash contains the COX-2 inhibitor Berberine and that COX-2 inhibitors are currently being touted as preventing or alleviating symptoms of alzheimer's, arthritis and colon cancer. It also contains chelerythine and nitidine. Chelerythine was cytotoxic in tumor tests and nitidine is highly cytotoxic in leukemia tests.[42] Prickly ash is also known as "toothache bark." Cayce often prescribed it for hygiene of the teeth and gums, but also made these broader comments:

FROM CAYCE READING 457-3
> The prickly ash bark is for the lacteal ducts and their activity in dissemination throughout the system."[43]

FROM CAYCE READING 2790-1
> The prickly ash bark is for the blood supply, as acted upon in the emunctory forces of the liver itself, proper.[44]

FROM CAYCE READING 1012-1
> The prickly ash bark acts directly with the activative forces in the liver itself, in the gall duct, and as a stimulant to the pancreas and spleen's activity.[45]

In the following case which combined dental hygiene with a general systemic toxemia, Cayce suggested a paste be made of prickly ash bark and salt, and applied to the gums. The oral treatment would disinfect both the teeth and the digestive tract.

FROM CAYCE READING 4283-2
> The toxins are not from the teeth entirely, see, these only add to the other toxins. It was first produced by that streptococci bacilli and that as is known in this plane as "flu." The reaction is ... from autointoxication from the intestinal tract where the system has been allowed to gather from those portions that which should be eliminated from the system ... For the specific condition use this: To three ounces of distilled water add one ounce of bark of prickly ash, reduce by simmering to two gills, and strain. Heat common salt and add until a thin mixture is made. Wash or rinse the mouth with this every third day for three to five treatments ...[46]

Cayce prescribed prickly ash bark in more than a hundred readings and in those preparations it was combined, as in Hoxsey's formula, with burdock forty-nine times.[47]

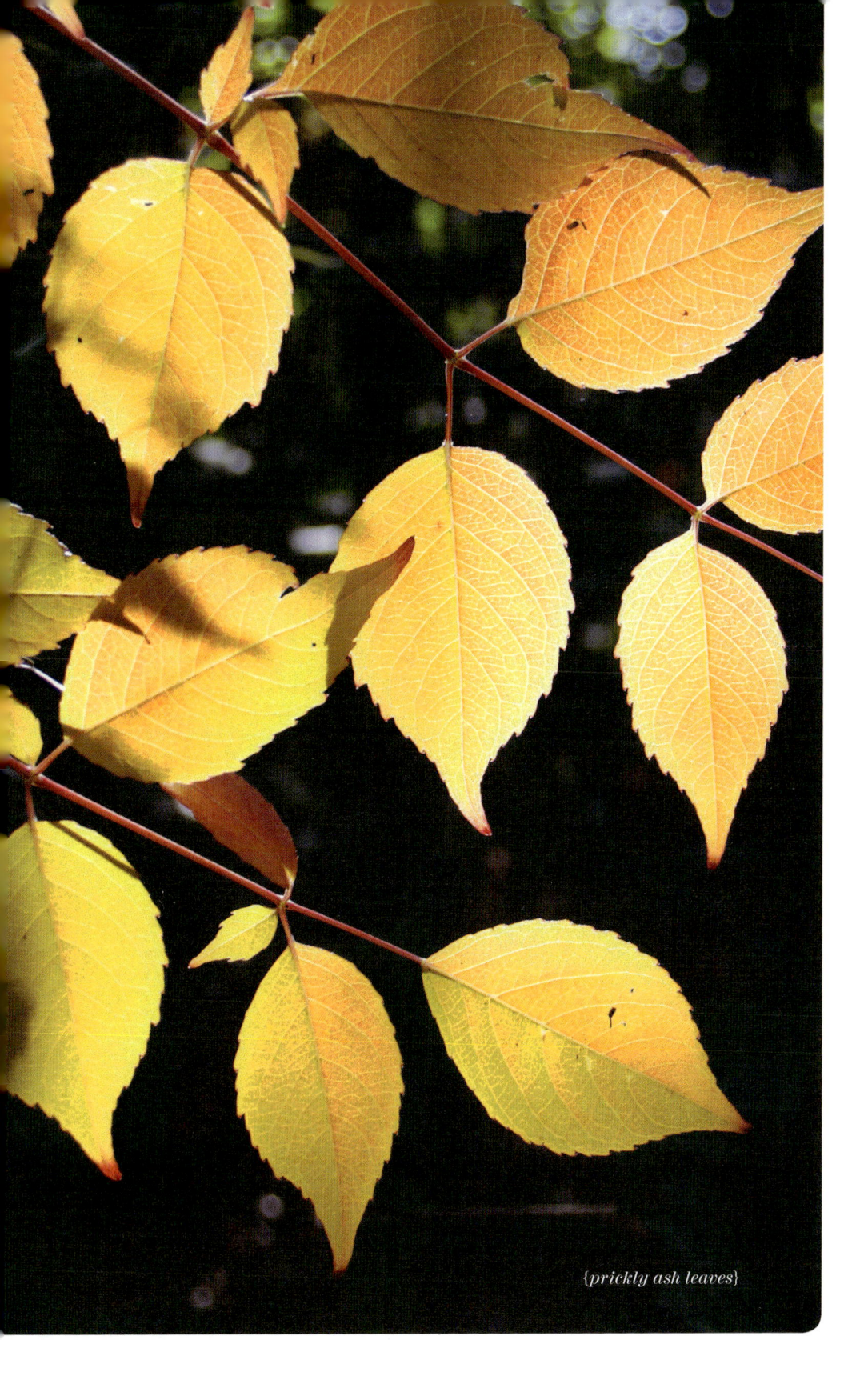

{prickly ash leaves}

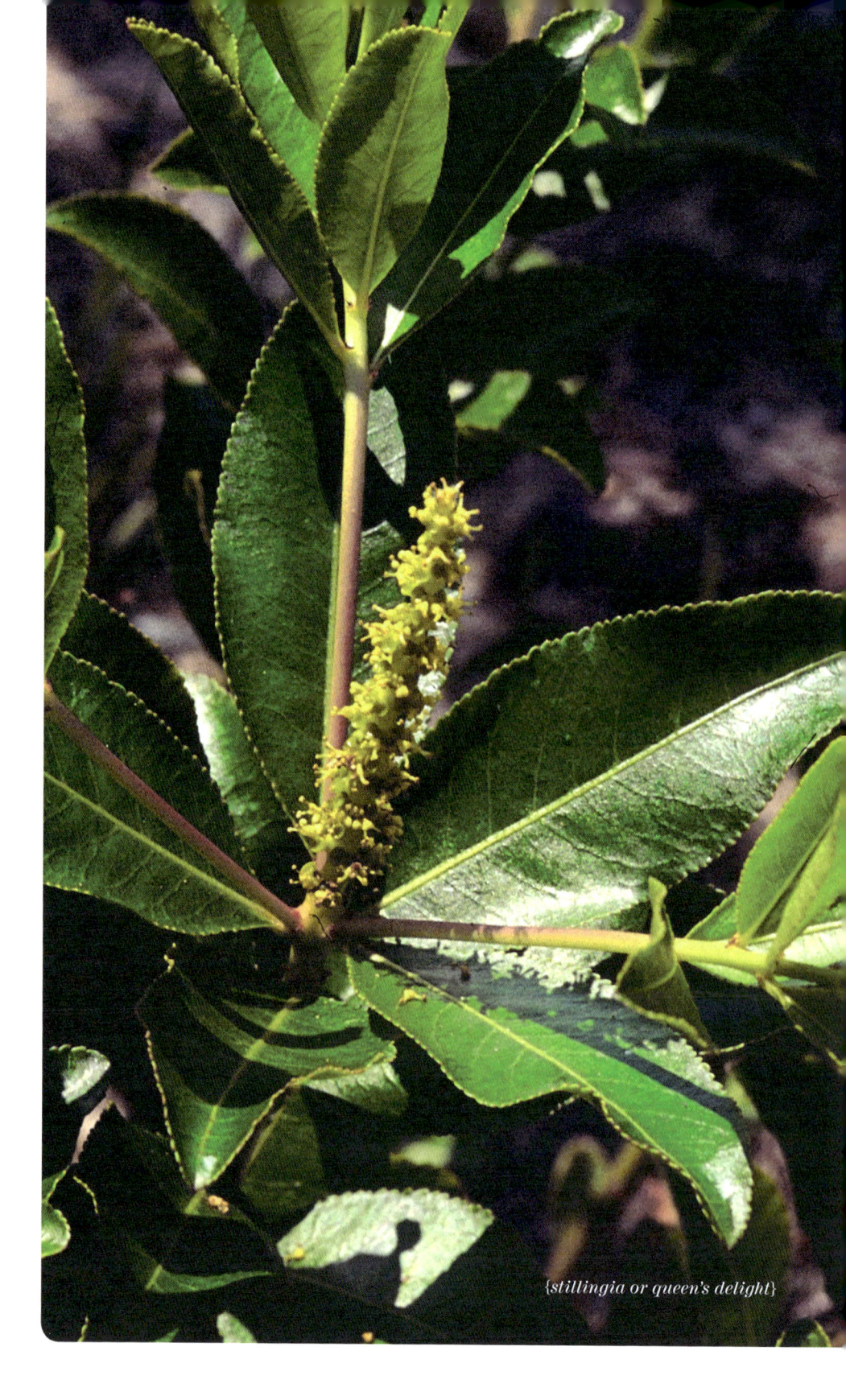

{*stillingia* or *queen's delight*}

Queen's Delight or Stillingia {*Stillingia sylvatica*}

Patricia Spain Ward's 1987 study, examining the history of the Hoxsey treatment for the OTA, indicated that German research in the 1980's had isolated two promising anti-tumor agents from the root of queen's delight or stillingia (as it will be referred to in this text).[48] NCI's Jonathan Hartwell mentions folkloric use of stillingia for carcinoma of the breast.[49] Eli Jones lists stillingia as an eclectic remedy for internal cancer.[50] Cayce recommended the use of stillingia in over 200 cases. He often related its use to liver function and eliminations. Interestingly, In fifty-nine cases he combined it with the Hoxsey formula ingredient, potassium iodide[51], which we will look at shortly.

FROM CAYCE READING 5509-1

Stillingia—an active force in the functioning of the liver, as related to the pancreas ... [52]

FROM CAYCE READING 5683-1

The stillingia is as a sedentary action for the glands of digestion, or the lacteals, with those that will make for a better coordination of the muco-membranes in the intestines, that will clarify poisons from the body.[53]

FROM CAYCE READING 404-4

Other properties; as in the stillingia, make for that activity with the pulsations between the liver, the heart, the kidneys, in such a manner as to still the circulatory forces there.[54]

Buckthorn {*Rhamnus cathartica*} and Barberry {*Berberis vulgaris*}

Of the nine herbs listed in the Hoxsey formula, two, buckthorn and barberry, were seldom used by Cayce. It is also known that Hoxsey occasionally added or removed ingredients from his formula.[55] For these reasons alone I will omit a detailed look at these two plants at this time. It should be noted, however, that both plants have historical medicinal use. Research suggests they also possess important anticancer compounds. In particular, the alkaloid berberine is found in barberry, and aloe-emodin and kaempferol are constituents of buckthorn.[56] An in-depth review of research concerning these compounds can be found in John Boik's excellent textbook, *Cancer and Natural Medicine*, listed in the Resources section of this book.

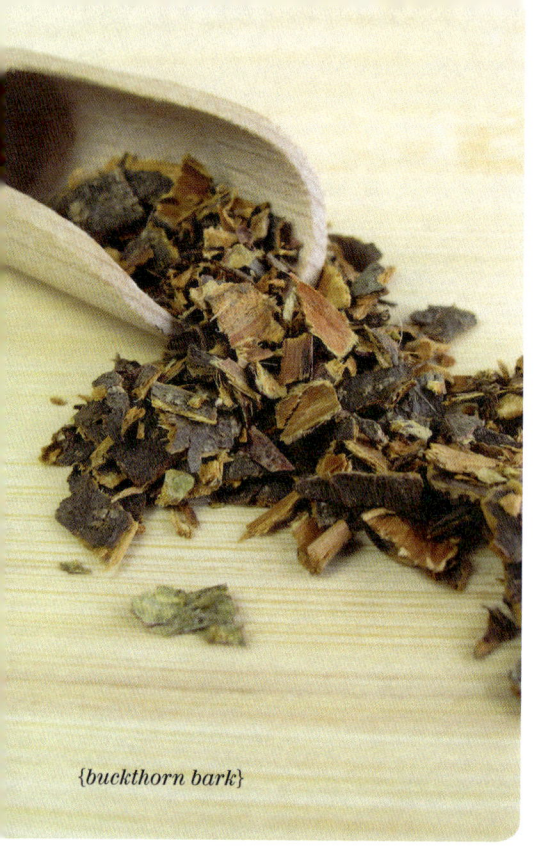

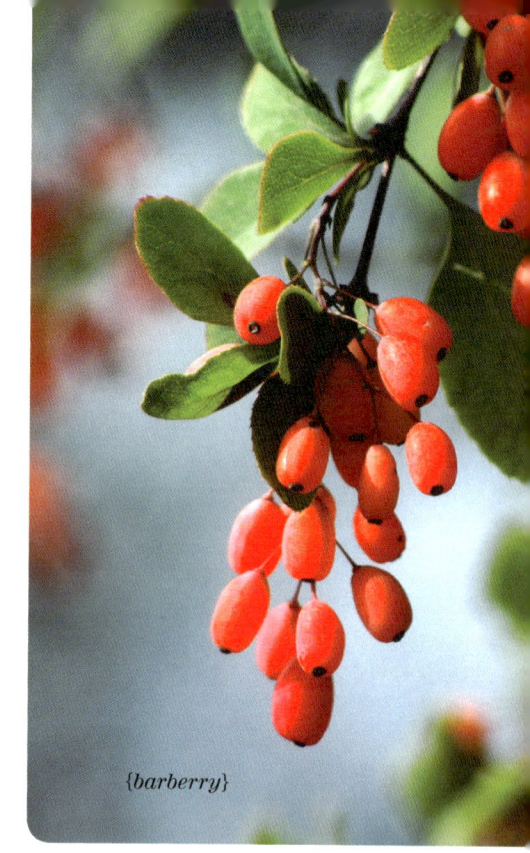

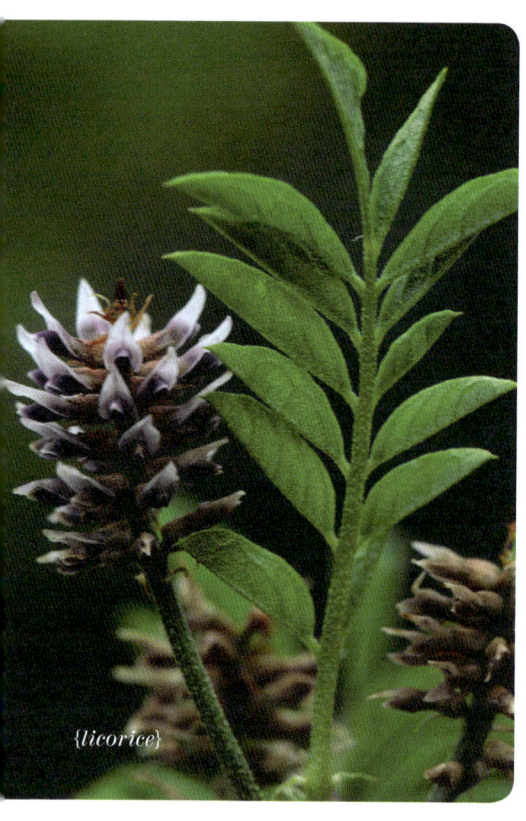

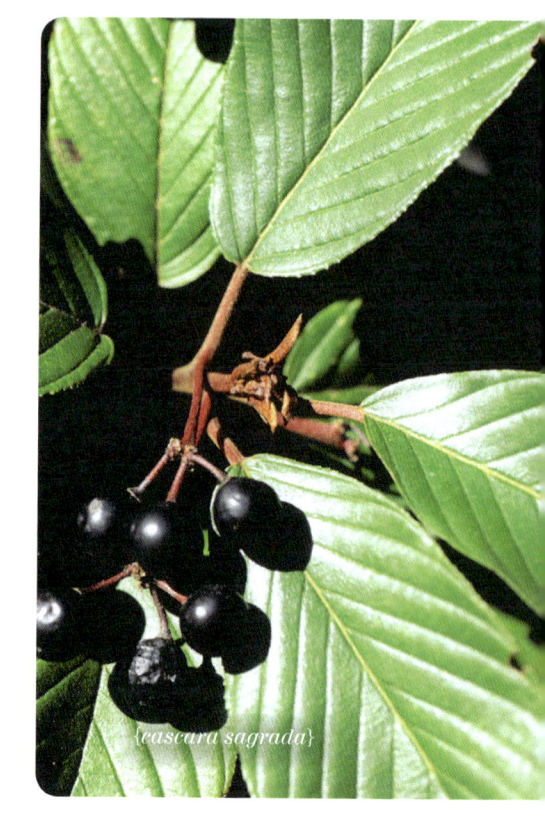

{buckthorn bark}

{barberry}

{licorice}

{cascara sagrada}

Licorice *{Glycyrrhiza glabra}* and Cascara Sagrada *{Rhamnus purshiana}*

The last two herbs of the Hoxsey tonic I want to consider are licorice and cascara sagrada. It is worth noting that Cayce not only used cascara sagrada and licorice often, but in a majority of cases he used them together.[57]

> **FROM CAYCE READING 4264-1**
>
> The action of these medicinal properties is given here to produce the proper equilibrium ... the licorice is an active principle, ... the active principle in the licorice to the blood supplying forces as they are taken from the system in the duodenum and through the liver here ... being active for new blood, ... with the licorice the cascara is to produce not an excitement of the mucous tissues of the stomach and intestines, but a condition that will act with these to eliminate through the proper channels the poisons now being absorbed by the blood back to the system ...[58]

Licorice was suggested in more than sixty Cayce readings and in more than forty of these, cascara sagrada was in combination with it.[59]

Cascara sagrada has primarily been used in herbal medicine as a laxative, containing aloe-emodins and cascarosides to stimulate elimination. It is also antiseptic, antibacterial, and antimutagenic. For patients with sensitive digestive systems, the Bio-Medical Center uses a modified Hoxsey formula including lactate of pepsin and reportedly reducing other herbs, including cascara sagrada.[60]

Licorice, like every other member of this herbal combination, has significant medicinal folk history and modern medical interest. Hartwell lists a page of reported uses of licorice, including tumors of the bladder, breast, stomach, cervix, liver, mouth, spleen and uterus.[61] Research in the year 2000 found that licorice components apigenin, kaempferol and salicylic acid-are COX-2-Inhibitors and have preventive effects on colon cancer. James Duke lists licorice as antiangiogenic, anticarcinomic, antimetastatic, antimutagenic, antinitrosaminic, antitumor, antioxidant, and antiinflammatory. He also notes that research showed that licorice component, glycyrrhizic acid, inhibited activity in a human colon tumor cell line.[62]

Licorice has long been used by herbalists to sooth internal inflammation, reduce bacteria, and promote elimination and immune function. Licorice has extensive use in European and Asian herbal tradition.

Potassium Iodide

The final Hoxsey ingredient is not an herb at all, but a compound of iodine and potassium. Potassium iodide has been a standard treatment for syphilis in this century. It has been used successfully to eliminate cancerous tumors in veterinary medicine.[63] It was distributed by the government, both in this country and in the Soviet Union following nuclear power plant-disasters, to nearby residents to reduce the incidence of thyroid cancer.[64]

Potassium iodide was suggested by Cayce on more than 200 occasions[65] and often in herbal formulas very similar to Hoxsey's. In the following case of a woman suffering hallucinations and about to be committed to a mental hospital, Cayce found lesions in the pineal and pituitary glands, resulting from pressures during an earlier pregnancy as well as distress to pelvic nerves from physical pressure and toxins in the blood.

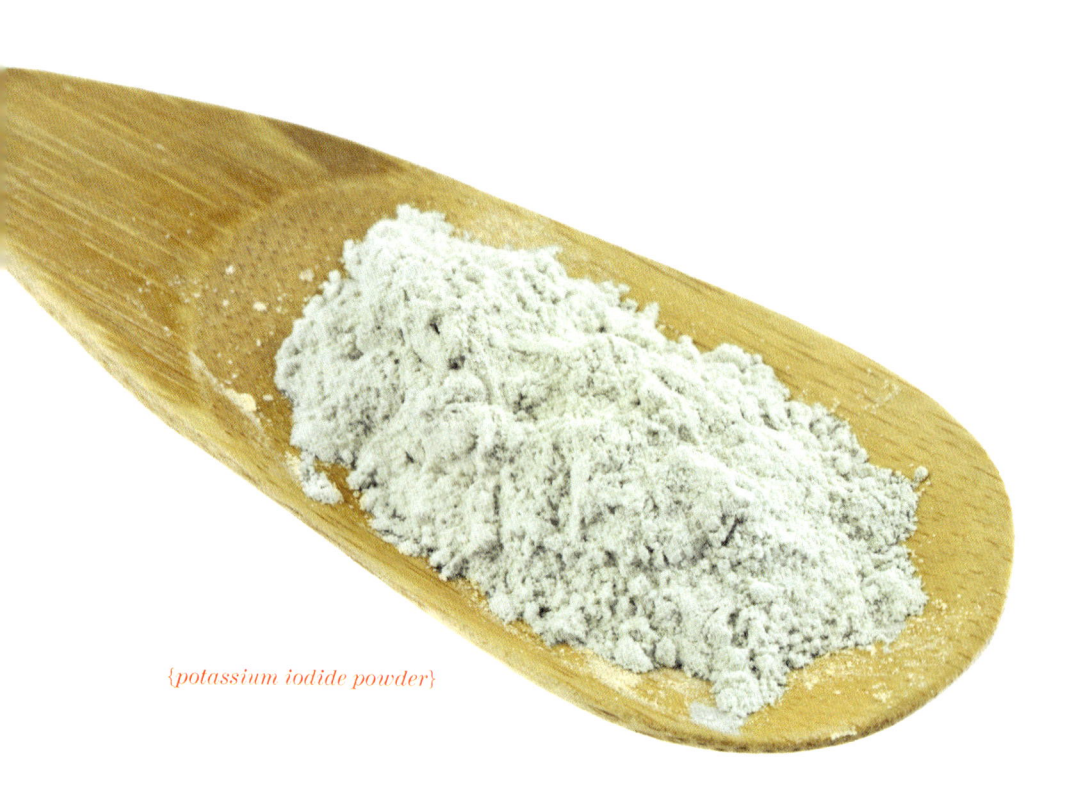

{potassium iodide powder}

FROM CAYCE READING 3996-1

Then to bring the normal conditions for this body, while it will take care and attention, and be hard to do, ...this may be accomplished with persistence, and consistent use of these properties for the body ...

fluid extract yellow dock root	½ ounce
fluid extract burdock root	½ ounce
fluid extract stillingia	½ ounce
fluid extract poke root	¼ ounce
iodide of potassium	30 grains
simple syrup sufficient to make	6 ounces

Dose would be half a teaspoonful twice each day.[66]

Finally, in a case involving nerve impairment and blood toxicity, Cayce gave this formula, again very similar to Hoxsey's formula, and again containing potassium iodide.

FROM CAYCE READING 4697-1

fluid extract of wild cherry	½ ounce
fluid extract of yellow dock root	½ ounce
fluid extract of burdock root	½ ounce
fluid extract of poke root	½ ounce
fluid extract of stillingia	½ ounce
iodide of potassium	½ ounce
simple syrup sufficient to make	8 ounces

Shake solution well together. The dose would be ½ teaspoonful four times each day. Let one of the doses come just at retiring, the others before meals. When all the quantity is taken, take the adjustments. We will bring the body to its normal condition and forces.[67]

Conclusion

Hundreds of patients have testified in court that the herbal formulas of naturopath Harry Hoxsey cured them of cancer. Edgar Cayce suggested formulas almost identical to those of Harry Hoxsey in some cases of cancer. For those familiar with Cayce, this strongly supports the synergy and chemical effectiveness of Hoxsey's herbal therapy. Both historical records and modern research affirm the promise of these herbal ingredients, particularly in anticancer or general detoxification therapies. Often, people aware of the medical information in the Edgar Cayce readings have difficulty applying it. We no longer have Edgar to give "check readings". Mechanical equipment and ingredients no longer exist, or have changed in manufacture. Pharmacies are unable to prepare the formulas. Having experienced these limitations myself, my excitement was increased in finding the original Hoxsey formula still manufactured and administered. It is reasonable to assume that some ingredient variability has occurred over time. Yet, with Mildred Nelson and staff personally administering the therapy until her recent passing, and with the medical staff unchanged, continuity and quality control should still exist. Mildred's sister, Liz Jonas, now oversees the Bio-Medical Center operation. This therapy provides a conveniently available, professionally administered, alternative therapy for patients with cancer.

When I think back to my own family's illness, I know it would have been difficult to consider traveling to Mexico for medical help. And yet it was physically as easy as traveling to San Diego and taking public transit. Several DVDs now available from different producers view the clinic operation and demonstrate its ease of access.

The real barrier for many in using this or any alternative herbal therapy has to do with legitimate skepticism in the value of the therapy. Noting the important difference between cynicism and skepticism, Edgar Cayce, in his readings, praised healthy skepticism as the mark of the true seeker. It is my hope that this book will be of help to those seeking medical options for treating cancer. The broader goal has also been to demonstrate that in fact the medicine is all around us. Benefiting from the courage of Harry Hoxsey and the extraordinary gifts of Edgar Cayce, we now have an even clearer picture of how to create life saving detoxifying medicine from nature. In the vision presented in the Revelation, the leaves of the tree of life bring healing to the nations. May our world realize this vision as we learn to recognize and apply nature's healing gifts.

{sassafras tree}

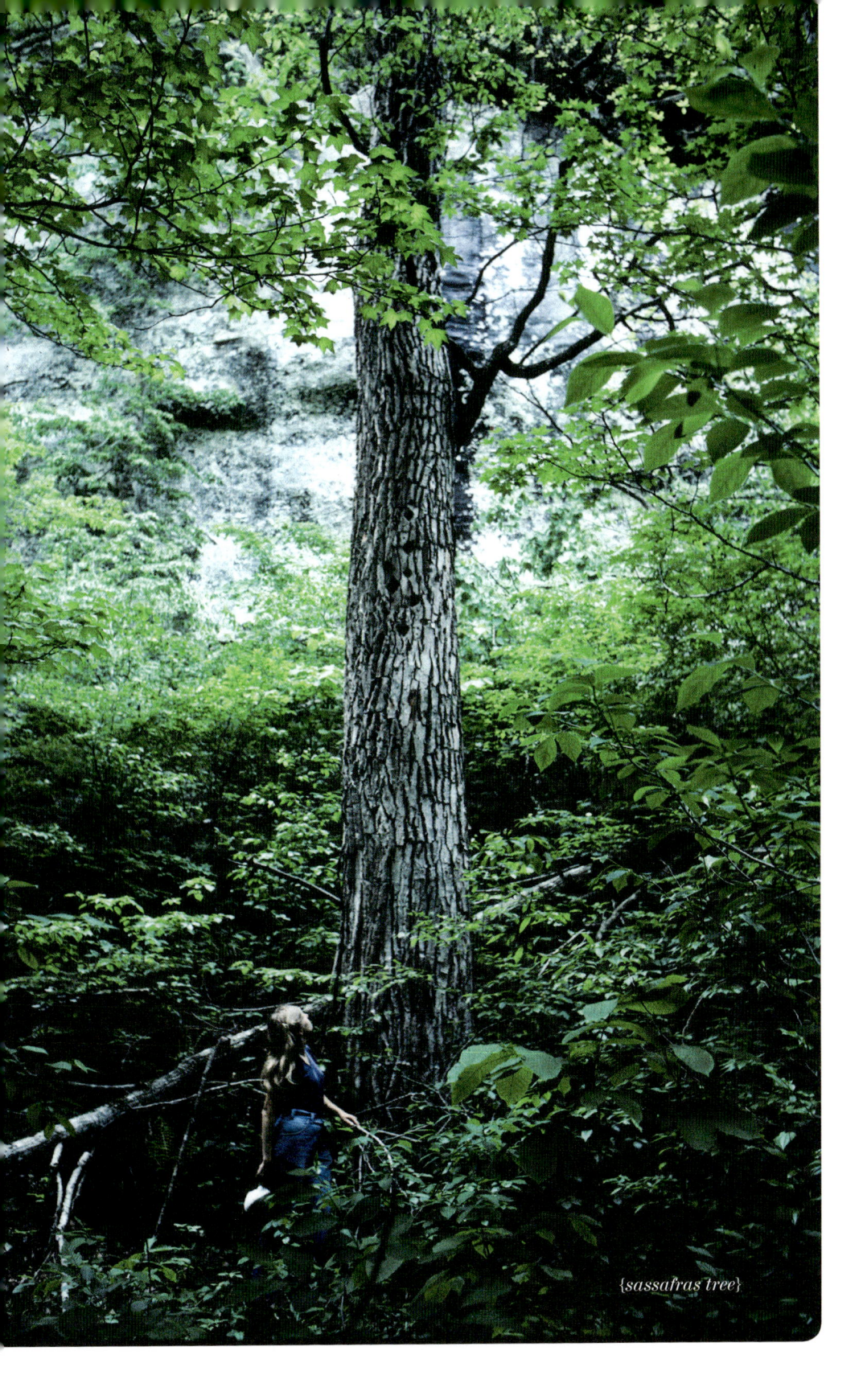

While in the waiting room of the C[...] patients, some new, some returning [...] (coming back once a year for a ph[...] negativity in that room. The smile[...] and the wonderful success stories in [...] truly one of the most uplifting exp[...] There was a book of [...] of our experience at the Clinic an[...] [...]hed to make about our cancer. [...] phone numbers in case anyo[...] [...] sure that the Lord was r[...]

Part III } Testimonial Correspondence

For more than fifty years, numerous testimonials have emerged concerning the successful use of herbal formulas similar to those of Edgar Cayce and Harry Hoxsey. The following stories are recent and from my own hometown. In a few cases they concern close friends and acquaintances. These letters are reprinted with the permission of the library of the Association for Research and Enlightenment (A.R.E.) in Virginia Beach, Virginia. They do not suggest that herbal medicine alone is a magic bullet which will always reverse cancer. The use of any medicine is but one important element within an individual's total healing environment. Its effectiveness will be influenced by other important factors, such as nutrition, rest and exercise, the use of supportive adjunctive therapies, work and home environments, mental attitudes and spiritual faith. Each case here represents one individual's unique healing path. I have edited for clarity and brevity, but have not altered the writing style or personal opinions expressed in these letters. Their honest depictions of fear, suffering, and courageous action illustrate, I believe, personal dimensions often lost in medical and political debates. I think you will agree that they are strongly suggestive of the potential power and sophistication of plant medicines in healing.

CASE ONE: UTERINE CANCER
BY SUSAN S. BAER

In October of 2002, I awoke in the middle of the night hemorrhaging. My husband took me to the emergency room at the Virginia Beach Hospital. They stopped the bleeding and sent me home with a gynecologist's name. I made an appointment and went to the gynecologists. He examined me and said he had never seen anything like my condition in all of his twenty some years in practice. He then sent me in for a sonogram. From there I was sent to Dr. Nasr, the oncologist, who scheduled me for an operation. After the operation, Dr. Nasr informed me that the cancer had gone from my uterus into an ovary and he had given me a complete hysterectomy. On my first appointment after the operation, I went into Dr. Nasr's office with my husband on one side of me and my daughter on the other holding me upright because I was so weak. Dr. Nasr informed me that I'd have to have a long series of chemotherapy treatments which I would begin immediately and turned me over to the nurse who explained exactly what I could expect.

When my little family arrived home that night, we were all in a very dejected mood. My daughter, Cheryl was very upset as she felt I was in such a weakened condition that I wouldn't make it through even one round of chemo. (The doctor had also said after chemo I would need radiation).

The next day Cheryl went to the A.R.E. Library in the hope of finding some help for me. She met a friend of hers who is the librarian (Linda Caputi) and told her about my bout with cancer. (Here is where the Lord stepped in) Linda said an airline pilot, Roger Bloom, had just published a pamphlet about the Hoxsey Formula and the Bio Medical Center in Tijuana, Mexico. (Roger's mother and father had both died of cancer before they had ever had the opportunity to hear of the Bio-Medical Center). When Roger had the opportunity to visit the center he was very impressed by the doctors and the patients and their testimonials on their successes in conquering their cancer. Cheryl happened to know Roger Bloom, as he was a dear friend, so she phoned him and his wife informed her that he was out of town but she knew of a local chiropractor who just got home from a trip to the Bio-Medical Center. Once again it turned out my daughter knew this chiropractor, so she called her and made an appointment for us to visit her. She told us of her uplifting experiences at the Center and loaned us some tapes of patients testimonials about the help they had found at the Center. She also explained how they work with diet, vitamins and the herbal formula that is the main component of the therapy.

When I, along with my husband and daughter, returned to Dr. Nasr's office and told him I was going a different route and wouldn't be taking chemo or radiation he was very upset and told us if I went for the alternative treatment, I would be back within three months begging for the Chemotherapy.

Cheryl got her and I airline reservations and we flew to San Diego around the thirteenth of December. When we arrived in California, we got a shuttle from the airport to the car rental agency and drove from there to the

International Motel in San Ysidro (outside of San Diego). We informed them at the Motel that we wanted to go to the Bio-Medical Center. They said the shuttle would be there at 8 a.m. the following morning.

We were taken to the clinic, arriving there about 8:45 a.m. Upon arriving, I signed in as a new patient and gave them all documents from doctors and my hospital pertaining to my cancer (x-ray, M.R.I., C.T. scan and my oncologist and family doctor's comments). I was given a gown to put on and asked for a urine specimen. They took a pelvic and chest x-ray. They took my blood pressure, temperature, weight and measured my height Then Dr. Polacios, who was a member of their medical staff, gave me the most extensive physical I have ever had. Then I was told to get dressed and if I wished, have lunch at the small restaurant connected to the clinic while Dr. Polacios studied my tests. When she was through she would call me into her office.

When Dr. Polacios called me, she said it was possible I might have another tumor on my sacrum. She suggested when I arrived back in Virginia Beach, I should find a doctor who wasn't adverse to working with alternative treatments of cancer and if I did have another tumor as they suspected I should have a series of intravenous medications. (She gave me the names and amounts of the medications I would need). I was given six bottles of the Hoxsey Herbal Formula and three months supply of yew needles, (which I needed to take two capsules of three times a day) and a list of vitamins and a very strict diet I had to follow. They told me to come back in three months.

While in the waiting room of the Clinic, I looked at the patients, some new, some returning after many years (coming back once a year for a physical). There was no negativity in that room. The smiles, the looks of hope, and the wonderful success stories in fighting cancer. It was truly one of the most uplifting experiences of my life. There was a book of testimonials in which we could write of our experience at the Clinic and any comments we wished to make about our cancer. Some patients had left their phone numbers in case anyone wished to call them. (I felt sure that the Lord was right there in the midst of us.)

We left the clinic in the shuttle about 3 p.m. in the afternoon. That was the beginning of my road back to good health.

One other thing I would like to mention was that my blood marker before my operation was 73, and after my operation it was 82. When I returned to the clinic three months later my blood marker was around 6 and has remained there for the last four-and-a-half years. 0 to 30 is a normal blood marker for uterine cancer. Also, when I arrived back in Virginia Beach and found a doctor that wasn't adverse to working with alternative treatments, it was discovered I didn't have another tumor. God is good!

{axus baccata or common yew}

CASE TWO: BREAST CANCER
BY BARBARA F. SIKES

It was September 16, 2002 that I was diagnosed with breast cancer – intraductal carcinoma was the official designation on the pathologist's report. I'd had it sent to be read by a second pathology lab just to be sure it was accurate. It was confirmed. A very scary two days ensued. I say two days because it was just two days later that I attended a Holistic Health Symposium for which I'd already registered. As a chiropractor I like to keep up with the latest in alternative and complementary medicine. At that symposium I learned about the Hoxsey Clinic, or Bio-Medical Center, as it is now called.

Thirty years earlier, in September of 1972, I had been diagnosed with multiple sclerosis. At the time there were no conventional treatments for MS—only medicines like prednisone that were supposed to help with the symptoms. In a way I was fortunate to learn after a few doses of prednisone that my body was much sicker with it than without it. That forced me to begin to look elsewhere—beyond what conventional doctors were offering —for MS treatments. I was fortunate to learn about the work of Dr. Roy Swank and his research with MS since the late 1940's using a very low saturated fat diet as a treatment for MS. I had nothing to lose and could see it was a healthy diet, so went on it. Within four years the MS had stabilized and I still follow it now after thirty-five years. I am blessed to be doing really well in spite of an MS diagnosis. During those years I went back to school to get my doctorate in chiropractic and my journey into alternative health care became well established.

So in 2002, when I was now faced with a cancer diagnosis, I'd been dealing with an auto immune disorder (MS) for all these years, and was scared—to be honest—to submit myself to surgery, chemo and/or radiation. What would that do to my system? Two or three doses of prednisone had made me sick—how would my system handle the much stronger and more toxic drugs of chemotherapy? But I didn't know enough about alternative cancer treatments to feel comfortable, let alone confident, about *not* doing conventional treatments.

So in the two days following my learning of the diagnosis, I attended the symposium and by Divine Synchronicity, two of the presentations that year were on cancer, and one of them was about Harry Hoxsey, his herbal treatments for cancer and the clinics he had started. After almost forty years in this country, they moved to Mexico in 1963. So by 2002 they had an almost eighty-year track record. I began further research and talked to patients all over the world who had been to the clinic up to twenty-eight years earlier and were still going strong. I watched the video, read the books and was down there in two weeks. I had also researched a few other possibilities in this country—one in particular down in Texas. They would charge $450 for the doctor to review records, $750 to see the doctor personally, and $4,500 a *month* to begin the treatments (This was in 2002). By comparison, the Bio-Medical Center charged $3,500 for *life.* You are asked to pay a third on each of your first three visits. No bills are ever sent. You are also asked to pay for any additional tests on each visit.

While it was all new and far away from where I lived on the east coast, the trip was pretty easy. I flew to San Diego and stayed in a motel in San Ysidro, California which provided shuttle buses to and from the clinic in Mexico. Any anxiety was allayed once I got there. The doctors and staff were so professional and friendly. The other patients were very encouraging to newcomers and it was reassuring to hear their stories. I was given a thorough exam, along with blood tests and urinalysis. X-rays were taken. I was then called back in to the doctor's office to go over their findings and make the recommendations. For me that included the herbal tonic to be taken four times daily along with dietary restrictions and other supplements. I was then sent home and asked to return in three months, which I did. Gradually the visits were extended to every six months and since 2005 I've just returned yearly. The tumor had been monitored physically and with blood tests. In 2004 one of my doctors in the U.S. requested I get a PET scan—it showed "minimal activity" in the affected breast and stated it was "within normal limits". I was on the right track! In 2005, new diagnostic equipment became available at the clinic which is able to distinguish between healthy and cancerous tissue. That was the first year I had a specific measurement of what was left of the tumor. When repeated in 2006 the test showed that the tumor was even smaller, and when I returned in 2007 there was no more evidence of any cancerous tissue! However, I plan to stay on the same treatment routine for at least another year to reconfirm the results, and before discontinuing the tonic. The dietary restrictions, as with those for the MS, have become routine and I can't imagine changing those to any great degree.

Additionally, I must stress the importance of the following components in this approach to cancer (or any) treatment. Getting plenty of rest, dealing with stress, keeping laughter, joy, and passion in your life, having a spiritual frame of reference, getting out in nature, and modest exercising all are critical adjuncts to the recovery process. For me that meant cutting back on work hours, continuing with meditation that I'd been doing for many years, taking up walking, *dis*continue watching the news, and expanding my already strong pull to spiritual studies.

UPDATED TESTIMONIAL: 2011 NON-CONVENTIONAL CANCER TREATMENT AT THE BIO-MEDICAL CENTER

Almost four more years have passed since I first wrote this. I'd like to give an update on what has transpired since. When I went to the clinic in 2008 I went earlier than usual, as I was accompanying another friend. However, it had been a difficult winter. I'd had a couple of really bad colds and I had cracked a rib about eight months before. I felt as if my immune system had been severely stressed. With all that going on I was not totally surprised when they found that the tumor had grown a little from the year before. What was so reassuring at this frightening turn of events was that the doctors, while taking it very seriously, seemed to know exactly what to do. My doctor adjusted her recommendations. They included adjusting the amount of tonic, the type and amount of supplements and home care, and incorporating a conventional prescription drug, taxus—which is a form of tamaxofin. I like the fact that they are not averse to using conventional therapies if indicated. The doctor also wanted me to return in six months rather than a year—which I was glad to do. On my return trip in October of 2008 we found the tumor shrinking again, and by 2010 there was once again no more evidence of cancer.

This whole episode confirmed to me that I had made the right choice. From my personal observation of the conventional world of treating cancer, patients go through the series of surgery, radiation and chemotherapy. Their immune system is weakened during the process with the hope being that the cancer will be killed without losing the patient. I have seen friends go through months if not years of hair loss, disruption to their whole digestive system, blood loss from the effects of chemo, recurrent hospitalizations, feeling fatigued or just crummy for days after each treatment and begin to rebound just in time for the next session (or onslaught). I know my choices aren't for everyone. Often over the years people have asked me, "Aren't you scared of not doing what the doctors say to do?" My response has always been, "No, the conventional stuff of getting cut on, radiated, and poisoned with chemo is much scarier!"

I haven't even mentioned the enormous financial burden these treatments leave with patents and families. Again, this is personal observation with individuals who already had decent insurance coverage, and still they are left with huge debts. Once more I am grateful that my choice has been infinitely less costly. Financially and every other way!

It's been ten years this year since the lump first showed up, and eight-and-a-half since the cancer diagnosis, and I'm still going strong. Thank you God. I am *so* grateful!

CASE THREE: PROSTATE CANCER
BY KARL STRACK

I was diagnosed with prostate cancer in January of 2006. I had a PSA (prostate-specific antigen) of 8.3 (under 4 is considered normal). It was biopsied for confirmation. I opted not to use a traditional method of treatment. I decided to go to the Hoxsey clinic in Mexico.

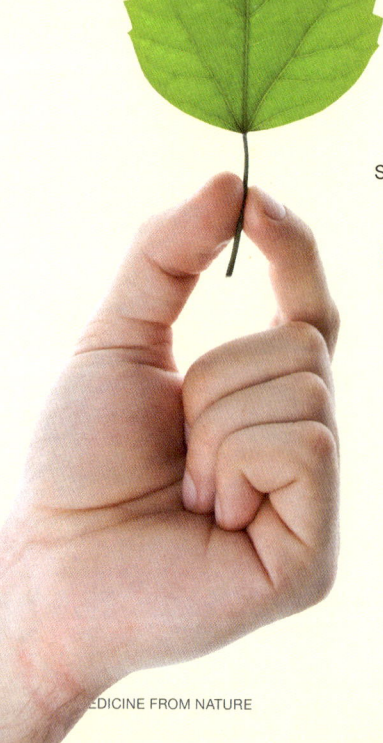

I was uncertain, nervous, and fearful before my first visit to the Hoxsey clinic. I was amazed at how kind and helpful the entire staff was. After testing, everyone goes to a waiting room and waits to discuss the results with a medical doctor. This waiting area provided an excellent opportunity to meet other patients and listen to their stories and discuss their various stages of recovery. I was just astonishing to see the immensely positive attitude of the patients as well as the entire staff, including the maintenance people. The entire attitude was about 'when I will be cured' not 'will I?'.

After what seemed like a lifetime, I was called in to talk with the doctor I was assigned to. The doctor talked with me for about two hours, discussing my regime and what I could expect.

I followed their instructions faithfully for several months, and then went back for my second visit. Again, I wound up in the waiting room after my exams, more nervous than the first time I was there. I met more people and again, they were very positive. I should note here that a lot of these people had advanced cancers and were told there was nothing more that could be done by their U.S. doctors. These people were improving! I was a little surprised at how open and eager everyone was to talk about their situation. I got the feeling like we were all part of a family pulling for each other. I was "finally" called in to see the doctor. After going over the test results, my program was modified slightly to reduce my cholesterol level. The results for my blood work would not be ready for several days, so I was asked to call back later in the week. The doctor wound up calling me and told me my PSA was 0.20. I was quite confused. I asked what kind of scale this was on and the doctor assured me that it was on the same scale as my original 8.3. It took several moments for me to grasp what I had just been told, and then I couldn't help just screaming for joy and then bursting out in tears.

Editor's Note: Prostate cancer patients receiving treatment at the Bio-Medical Center have reported the use of male hormone blocking drugs as recommended supplemental treatment to the standard Hoxsey herbal therapy. While such drugs do lower the patient's PSA test readings they may also create very undesirable side effects. If considering the use of hormone blocking drugs in prostate cancer recovery it is important for patients to be familiar with the possible negative effects of reduced testosterone. An easily understood explanation of the subject can be found in chapter twenty of the latest revision of Outsmart Your Cancer *by Tanya Pierce. Her book is in the Suggested Reading listings in the Resources section of this book.*

CASE FOUR: BREAST CANCER, SURGERY SUGGESTED
BY LINDA CAPUTI

Linda Caputi, a retired registered nurse, is on staff at the A.R.E. Library, and has been involved with the Cayce material for the last twenty-five years. She is the author of the book, Epilepsy—Jody's Journey: An Inspiring True Story of Healing with the Edgar Cayce Remedies.

A few years have gone by but I'm still in awe at how my daughter-in-law's experience with breast cancer unfolded and how God arranged all the synchronicities. God and all her angels!

Ever since I knew her, Socheata loved angels. Actually, angels and anything purple. It made it easy to find her an appropriate gift for birthdays or special events. She also loved my son, which was a good thing, because he loved her dearly. They married and soon had three children plus a growing business near Washington, D.C.

Since I live in Virginia Beach and work at the A.R.E. Library, I don't get to see them often. But Socheata sends frequent pictures of the grandkids and sometimes even of the grandkids' parents romping around as if they were the kids.

However, one day my son called me at work, upset. Socheata had gone to her physician about a lump in her breast. She was only thirty-two years old. I called her as soon as possible and she told me she had had the lump for a few months but thought it was just a painful pulled muscle—except it kept growing. Then one night, she had a vivid dream. In the dream she was told she had cancer and that it might kill her. Without delaying any further, she called her doctor for an appointment the next morning. After a very uncomfortable needle biopsy and a week's wait, the results came back positive for cancer.

Her doctor advised her she should begin with chemo right away, and then within a few weeks have a mastectomy. But Socheata had thought things over seriously and knew chemo wasn't something she would do. A mastectomy... well maybe.

Over the years, working at the A.R.E. has opened my mind to more modalities of healing than my nursing background had originally exposed me to: an array of Cayce's remedies of course (a healthy diet, castor oil packs, osteopathy, massage, prayer and meditation) plus other approaches such as Dr. Upledger and cranial sacral therapy, Mariel healing, Reiki, etc. In fact, I had become very familiar with Cayce's remedies for numerous ailments, including the remedies for epilepsy that had healed my daughter Jody and the ones for muscular dystrophy that had significantly helped me.

There were many Cayce readings on various types of cancer, including breast cancer, but what impressed me the most with its simplicity was a tonic consisting of a few well-known herbs.

Coincidentally, at an A.R.E. conference where Roger Bloom spoke, I learned that a man by the name of Harry Hoxsey had put together such a formula and had been treating thousands of people successfully for cancer in his clinics (from 1925 until 1960). Seventeen of these clinics were operating throughout the United States at one time before the American Medical Association, through the FDA, closed him down. Hoxsey sued and won but decided against reopening and facing further harassment.

Instead, his longtime nurse opened one last clinic in Tijuana, Mexico. Thankfully, that clinic, the Bio-Medical Center, is still operating today using the same herbs that Cayce recommended.

A number of people I've known had gone to the clinic and were healed of cancer—prostate, Hodgkin's lymphoma, ovarian and breast cancer (both women with breast cancer were advised that in their case a mastectomy would not be necessary). So when Socheata told me about her diagnosis, I shared with her what I had learned about Hoxsey and suggested that she visit the clinic for a consultation.

To my great relief, she agreed, and within a few days Socheata and my son were on a flight to California.

They would check in at a hotel in San Diego where most visitors to the clinic stayed, and the next morning be picked up by a van which would then take them (and any other new and repeat patients) for the forty-five minute drive into Tijuana. At the end of the day, they would be taken back to their hotel by the same van, and that would complete their visit to the clinic.

Later on, Socheata related to me how surprised she was at the attitude of the patients in the van and clinic—everyone seemed truly happy and cheerful, though it was early morning and breakfast would have to wait until after blood tests would be drawn. The staff was also very kind and professional and spoke English well, though many languages could be heard because of the diversity of people who came from all over the world.

After their arrival at the clinic, which was a lovely older mansion, everyone waited together for their turn to be seen by the medical doctors. Joyful greetings among clients who knew each other from former visits and conversations among new ones passed the time.

My son and daughter-in-law started talking to a woman who sat by herself near them. She too was American. It was her third visit back, and she had only good things to say about her experience there.

"So how did you find out about the clinic?" the woman asked my son.

"Oh, my mother told us about it." he answered.

"And how did you learn of the clinic?" my son asked her.

"There was a woman in a library who told me about it after I told her I had been diagnosed with breast cancer about a year ago."

"The Edgar Cayce Library?" my son carefully inquired.

"Yes, exactly!" she said, surprised, "How did you know?"

"Well, that woman in the library is my mother." he told her, as they all laughed!

Later that night the three of them went to dinner together and called me in Virginia Beach to let me know how things had gone.

Their new acquaintance, whose name they mentioned but I didn't recall, had done well with her check-up and was told to continue with the Hoxsey tonic and the recommended diet (similar to Cayce's).

However, after the doctors consulted with each other—as they do for each client, Socheata was told to start with the tonic for the time being, and in her particular case, arrange for a mastectomy as soon as possible. The tumor was large, attached to her chest wall and causing her to be anemic.

This wasn't what Socheata and my son wanted to hear but they appreciated what they had been told. They had also learned at the clinic that occasionally, in advanced cases, the doctors recommended low doses of chemotherapy if they felt it was called for in order to give a person the extra time for the tonic to work. But the doctors had not told Socheata to start chemo—and there was no way she would have anyway.

{buckthorn oil}

Disappointed, my son and Socheata returned home. They had hoped surgery wouldn't be necessary, but that was not the clinic's opinion.

Socheata started on the Hoxsey tonic (and a number of supplements and diet the clinic recommended), but knew what she had to do if she wanted to live. She called her doctor for the name of a surgeon and set up an appointment to be seen.

That's when life got a-hell-of-a-lot more complicated.

When she went for her appointment, the surgeon told her, in no uncertain terms, he wouldn't do a mastectomy without her first having chemo!

"Well," she thought, "If he won't, I'll just find a surgeon who will."

She called her regular doctor and asked for other referrals but he warned her that she was going to run

48 • CANCER MEDICINE FROM NATURE

into the same issue. "They" don't do a mastectomy without first doing chemo or radiation.

Socheata called them all. And all said the same thing. More than a week or two had passed since their trip to the clinic by now.

My son called at work and told me their dilemma. They didn't know if Socheata would have to go to another country in order to find the right surgeon. "Do it my way or you don't get it done," seemed to be the attitude. Very frustrating and stressful, to say the least.

I hung up the phone, lost in thought, when it rang again.

It was a library patron from Arizona wanting to renew her overdue books. The woman said she was sorry that they were late but she had just gotten out of the hospital. I said I hoped she was better and then, on an impulse, asked if she knew any surgeons who would do a mastectomy without first doing chemo or radiation.

She suggested I contact Dr. Bill or Dr. Gladys McGarey—which I thought was a good idea, something I could do on my lunch break. I thanked her for her suggestion and we said good-by.

During the phone call, I had noticed a young woman standing nearby looking at some books. Now tentatively she walked over to me.

"I couldn't help but overhear your conversation just now. Maybe I can help. You see, my mother had the same problem a few years ago when she was diagnosed with breast cancer. She wanted a mastectomy but not everything else that came with it. She was going to use natural alternatives and change her diet, but wanted the tumor removed. Eventually she found a wonderful man who would do it.

"I have the name of the doctor if you'd like it," she said as she handed me a piece of paper with his name on it. "He's located somewhere in Richmond."

I think I just stared for a while at this angel in disguise before I could speak. "How can I ever thank you?" I finally said. "I'll follow up on this right away."

I asked how her mother was doing. "Very well," she replied. But when I inquired, the daughter wasn't sure of the specific remedies her mother had used (something else for me to look into another time). And soon after, she turned and left the library, leaving me slightly dazed.

It was quiet so I decided to take a quick look on the internet. There in black and white was the surgeon's telephone number. He was real, at least.But not wanting to give my daughter-in-law any false hope, I called the office to confirm what "the angel" had told me. Within moments I was put through to the surgeon's assistant—who did exactly that. She even said Socheata could be seen within the week!

I couldn't get off the phone fast enough to call Socheata and give her the information. She was as surprised as I had been and said she would call the office right away.

Later, after work, Socheata called me at home. They had made an appointment a couple of days away, and arranged for their children to be picked up from school. They would travel to Richmond in the morning (about a three-hour drive), see the surgeon, and be back in time for dinner.

Socheata was going to Richmond but still wasn't completely sure about the mastectomy. Maybe it wasn't necessary and the herbal tonic could take care of the tumor? And then again, why go through the pain and expense of surgery if she would die anyway?

Speaking about pain, let me digress for a moment: Socheata had been in pain for a couple of months by now, right where the tumor was located. Not unbearable, but painful nonetheless. However about four days after starting the tonic she told me that the pain had gone!

In any case, I prayed for Socheata to make the right decision for herself, whatever it was.

The day of the appointment my son and Socheata left early in case they got caught in traffic. But there was none and now they had time to spare. They located the doctor's office easily enough and then drove around in the neighborhood. There was a mall so they decided to park and go window shopping.

At one point as they walked, my son said to Socheata, "Doesn't that woman at a distance look like the woman we met at the clinic?"

"No, it couldn't be her, what would she be doing here?"

Not bothering to walk any closer they continued on their journey and leisurely returned to the doctor's office.

They met and liked the surgeon who explained the procedure and what to expect before and after. Despite lingering reservations, they decided to go ahead and schedule a date for surgery. They could always cancel if need be—but at least they had found a surgeon who would perform the mastectomy!

They drove back home and arrived in good time.

Later that evening the phone rang. It was the woman they had met at the clinic. They had given her their number when they left and thought nothing more about it.

"Oh, how nice," Socheata thought, "She's calling to say 'Hello'."

They chatted briefly before Socheata was taken aback by what the woman had to say.

"I really called because a funny thing happened today. I could have sworn I saw you and your husband when I went to a local mall on my lunch break."

"That was us!" Socheata said in disbelief. "We were early for an appointment to see a surgeon in Richmond, Dr..."

"What a coincidence! He's my surgeon and I think he's just terrific."

That was the finishing touch.

More than enough synchronicities occurred to convince the most skeptical mind and help Socheata come to peace with a disturbing decision that needed to be made.

Socheata went ahead and had surgery, without incident. She is doing beautifully and discontinued taking the Hoxsey tonic last year.

CASE FIVE: HODGKIN'S LYMPHOMA
BY DR. ALLEN S. CHIPS, D.C.H., PH.D.

The following paragraphs are excerpted with permission from an article in the April 2006 issue of Venture Inward Magazine. *The author, Dr. Allen S. Chips, D.C.H., Ph.D., has since published a detailed account of his healing in a book entitled* Killing Your Cancer Without Killing Yourself, *from Transpersonal Publishing.*

As an alternative health professional, I never thought I would be the one telling about my own battle with cancer. I'd helped others cure theirs, but did not expect to be in the position of needing the advice, "Physician, heal thyself." We always think that it won't happen to us—we take so many supplements, do our spiritual work, meditate, try to eat right, then *whammo!* the body does things that we don't consciously want. Like me, many embark upon a grand educational journey through alternative or allopathic medicine, in search of healing.

I came down with the first symptoms of night sweats and week-long fevers on Good Friday, in April 2003; was diagnosed with Hodgkin's lymphoma on May 21, right on my twentieth wedding anniversary; and reluctantly set up my first chemo date for June 16. My diagnosis was stage 2B—two areas of the body, traveling in the blood. Two tumors on the neck, four tumors between the heart and lungs, and growing. I was supposed to take twelve treatments of A.B.D.V. chemotherapy, with a PET scan after eight treatments, to determine whether chemo would be enough. If not, radiation would also be necessary.

I got on the recovery warpath in May by spending every day, from 7:30 a.m. to sometimes as late as 1 or 2 p.m., researching cures in a book or on the phone. I contacted a wide variety of treatment programs, oncologists, cancer researchers, alternative health practitioners, psychics, ministers, recovered cancer patients, and the National Institutes of Health's National Council of Complementary and Alternative Medicine (NCCAM).

My acupressure therapist gifted me with the booklet, *Cancer Medicine from Nature,* by Roger Bloom. The book made sense, as it emphasized the herbs Edgar Cayce recommended to rectify cancerous conditions. Herbal medicine made sense to me, as I recollected a Cayce reading suggesting there was a natural cure for every illness. I felt that God would have foreseen our conditions of illness and given us this grace; so I wanted to find out more about it while at the A.R.E.

My focus was on herbs and diet. I wanted to see what Edgar Cayce recommended not just to prevent cancer, but cure it. I found multiple recommendations of burdock root, stillingia, yellow dock root, wild cherry bark, and potassium iodide. I also found elderflower and noticed that Cayce recommended an alkaline diet.

Then I watched the video called *Hoxsey's Bio-Medical Center: The Experience,* which described a patient's experience at the clinic. A husband and wife who both recovered with the clinic's treatments produced it.

She'd been diagnosed with pancreatic cancer and given three months to live—twenty years ago! I later found out that typically those who are diagnosed with pancreatic cancer are told to skip chemotherapy because it would just shorten their lives. Traditional medicine offered no hope. Wow! I later phoned her to find out her husband was diagnosed with non-Hodgkin's lymphoma a few years after her cure, and he was also cured with Hoxsey therapy using no traditional medicine.

I took one round of chemo anyway, thinking I would do self-hypnosis and imagery to stave off the side effects. Afterward, I was anemic, had hives from an allergic reaction, severe, debilitating short-term memory loss (from intravenous steroids), blisters on my tongue, and the list goes on. I couldn't remember what I did or said from one moment to the next, and of all of my gifts from God, my mind is my most treasured asset. A few days later, when I went to church, my pastor looked at me and said, "What happened to you?" I told him that I took a chemotherapy treatment, and he said, "Maybe you needed to try it to find out it was something you should never do again." I agreed. I felt like death warmed-over, and I almost fainted a couple of times during the service.

In essence, I was on my own from here. I was a "no-show" on my next chemo appointment, and at my subsequent doctor's visit, my oncologist said I needed to have at least five more treatments (of twelve minimum) to have any remote chance of a cure. He recommended I take off from work for at least a year, close the speaking and publishing business, and have my wife support me. I said, "No way." He said, "You know one treatment won't cure you." I acknowledged that, and was officially signed off as "refusing treatment" in my medical charts. As I departed, I will never forget my oncologist's face as he shook my hand farewell, certain he would never see me again.

When I got to Tijuana on August 10, I requested an additional consultation with a homeopathic physician (all the physicians had been there fifteen to twenty years). In the waiting room, I read the visitor registry. It was filled with testimonials, many from patients who had returned for checkups many years later, still satisfied that the Bio-Medical Center had extended their lives. I read many stories of people whose cancer had metastasized but were cured with Hoxsey therapy in a last-ditch effort after traditional medicine had given up on them.

An oncologist who had worked at the clinic for eighteen years examined me. He said my liver and spleen were slightly enlarged, so we would need to stay in frequent contact to make sure the cancer was not spreading to my organs. Next I was shown all my CT scans, which covered a wall. The clinic's radiologist and several alternative medicine physicians pointed out cancer-related factors in the CT scans. That morning, I learned much more about the extent of my disease than I had in the U.S.

Later, I met again with my oncologist, who put me on a much stricter diet, eliminating pork, vinegar, tomatoes, processed sugar and flour, most fats, alcohol, and many preservatives. The diet added alkaline-forming foods, and took away acid-forming foods. Supplemental replacements were given for specific nutritional deficiencies. The premise for the diet, which had to be followed exactly, was that cancer couldn't grow in a highly alkaline environment. While stifling cancer growth it stimulated the immune system to attack the tumors. The herbs, which cleanse the blood and restore the organs, further boost the immune system and destroy the capillaries feeding the tumors, all of which was evidenced in my CT scans. Years on the diet rebuild the immune system to a level sufficient to prevent any cancers from recurring. The diet works like a vaccine. Once the immune system recognizes and overcomes certain cancer cells, the body maintains a permanent immunity to them.

Second, he put me on the "black tonic," as he called it. Their herbs were suspended in a potassium iodide base (instead of alcohol), which proved to be much more potent, as I would discover for the next two months while experiencing prolonged digestive tract cleansing. Apparently, the berberis, which is known for killing candida, was doing its job. Then, in the homeopathic consultation, I was put on two forms of Chinese medicine. The first was from Spring Wind Herbs, a Berkeley, California based Chinese medicine pharmacy that labeled the powdered tea, "Lymphoma Rx." The other was the new "miracle cure," as it's been referred to in the *International Journal of Oncology*, 2001, called Artemisinin. Nutracology in Hayward, California manufactures Artemisinin. It's a derivative of the herb *Artemesia* (sweet wormwood), which has been a long-time cure for malaria in Asia. An article written by Robert J. Rowen, M.D., stated that it's been credited with 100% effectiveness, in all cases studied, often resulting in complete remissions, but is not approved by the FDA. I was also put on Montana yew tree needles, the natural, much less toxic derivative of the popular chemo drug taxol.

The last phase was supplement education—keep taking CoQ-10, garlic, and multivitamins; stop the shark cartilage, and take coral calcium with magnesium instead, since it has several minerals our soil doesn't pass on to our foods anymore.

At the end of my consultation and examination, which cost less than $100, I was offered a lifetime supply of the herbal medicinal tonic. At that time, a patient could try the tonic for one year at a price of $700. Since I knew the remedy was going to work for me, and because the Bio-Medical Center recommended a minimum of five years on the tonic, I bought the lifetime supply.

My next visit was to our local hospital in November. The osteopath who examined the CT scan (on the screen in front of me, since he was my friend and neighbor) exclaimed, "These look necrotized! What have you been doing?" He knew I had given up chemo as soon as I started it, and he had been praying for me. I told him what I'd done to get to this point. Next, I flew out to Mexico for a checkup, and my Mexican oncologists said the same thing: "They (the tumors) look black, and small." Usually, it takes a year or so to boost the immune system high enough to kill and shrink the tumors to this degree, not three months!

In 2004, after two rounds of CT scans, one in the spring and one in the fall, I received a clean bill of health from my local traditional oncologist. He said, "You're done. You don't need to come back here anymore." He had become more interested in how I did it, so I promised him a lunch out after my one-year routine checkup due in the fall of 2005—when I would further explain these cures from nature.

Yes, the Bio-Medical Center doctors agreed, that the chemo was a help but not a cure; my traditional oncologist concurs. In fact, he originally believed it was a miracle from God. I believe it's a combination of the Cayce/Hoxsey herbs and alkaline diet, the daily imagery I utilized, and the people that God put in my path to teach me how to win the race. The A.R.E. introduced me to natural remedies I didn't realize existed. The Bio-Medical Center made available these unknown cures, and their holistic support system included a thorough education of diet, herbs, supplements, environment, and lifestyle factors. Throughout the process, they promptly responded to every email and phone call.

This journey made me realize that we are all on borrowed time, and we need to heed the saying *carpe diem,* which in Latin means, "seize the day." With gratitude, I owe my life and well being to Edgar Cayce, Harry Hoxsey, the people at A.R.E. and the Bio-Medical Center—and first and foremost, to God.

EDGAR CAYCE READING #2396-2

There is within the grasp of man all that in nature that is the counterpart of that in the mental and spiritual realms, and an antidote for every poison, for every ill in the individual experience, if there will but be applied nature, natural sources.

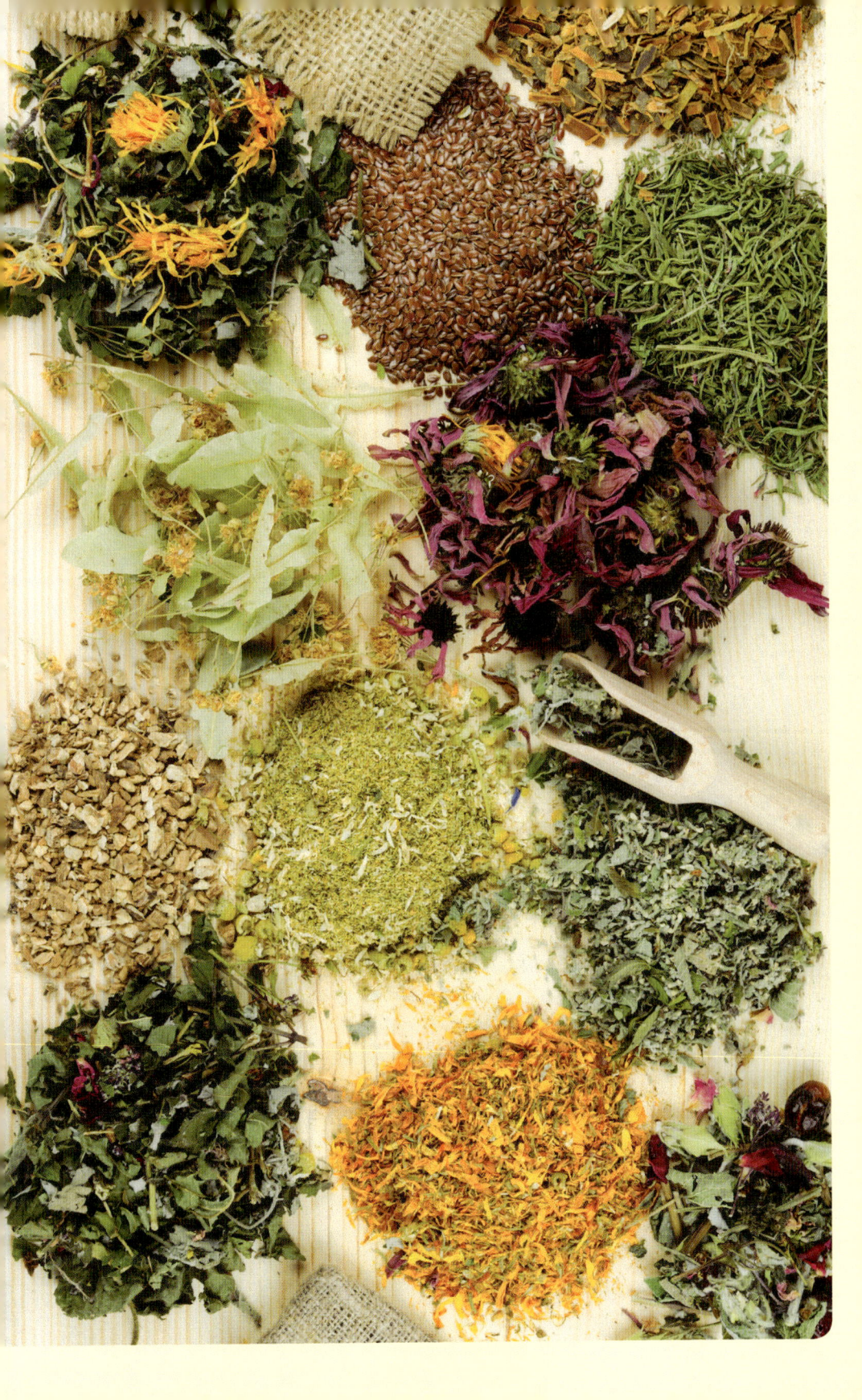

CASE SIX: BREAST CANCER
BY MYRNA

When I was diagnosed with breast cancer in November of 2000, I was shocked and upset. I was no different than anyone else regarding the "cancer" word. It strikes fear and dread in most people, especially when they are the ones who have it, and I was no exception.

My surgeon wanted me to decide what I wanted to do after the mastectomy—have reconstructive surgery with a plastic surgeon or leave it be. She was going on vacation, but said I should make an appointment for early January when she returned. In the meantime, I should talk to the oncologist, radiologist and plastic surgeon.

The radiologist wanted to nuke my lymph nodes, as well as the two tumors. The plastic surgeon not only wanted to reconstruct the breast to be removed, but also work on the good one so they would "match." The reconstruction would come from my lower abdomen—one side, anyway, and the other side would be removed so I would balance, and then would be discarded. Not a pretty picture.

When I saw the oncologist and told him I had to let the surgeon know what I wanted to do in the next two weeks, he said, "You don't have two weeks!!" That was December 4, 2000, only two weeks after the biopsy.

I was lucky. I have a friend who had cancer throughout her body in the early 1960's. She was given up to die by the doctors here in the U.S. The chiropractor she worked for bundled her up, and he and his wife took my friend down to Tijuana to the Bio-Medical Center. They told her she was so far gone, they were not sure she would make it, but they would give it all they had. At first, she could only keep down the Hoxsey tonic and carrot juice, but in eight months she was back on her feet and raising her two-year-old daughter. She is seventy-eight today and still free of cancer.

At first, I was going to have the surgery and then go down to the clinic to get rid of any lingering cancer cells. When I discussed it with my friend, she never told me what to do. Then, on my own, I realized that I was being foolish. If the tonic could kill the rest of the cancer lurking in my blood stream, it could certainly kill the tumors in the breast, without surgery, radiation or chemotherapy. December 6, 2000, just two days after seeing the oncologist and hearing his "death sentence," saying I didn't have two weeks, I was on my way to Tijuana and never looked back.

The line for new patients was very small, only a couple of us. The line for returning patients was practically out the door. That gave me encouragement. If they're returning, they must be getting good results.

The cancer was confirmed by the blood tests and I was given guidelines for a diet and a supply of tonic and yew tablets, which is the natural substance that forms tamoxafen—the breast cancer drug. The yew tablets would kill any stray cancer cells in the blood.

The diet consisted of no bleached flour, no white sugar, no sugar substitutes, no alcohol, no caffeine, no carbonated beverages, sea salt—no regular salt, no microwaving of food, and above all, nothing with vinegar or acetic acid and absolutely nothing with tomatoes, not even Mrs. Dash. The vinegar and tomatoes interfere with the tonic's effectiveness. So that meant no salad dressing, no mayonnaise, no BBQ sauce, no mustard, no catsup, no sauces, no spaghetti with tomato sauce, no tomatoes in my salad, etc. It was going to take a lot of will power and I thank God that I had it. The thought of the radiation, chemo, surgery and plastic surgery scared the living daylights out of me. After all, the graveyards are full of people who have been given those treatments and succumbed anyway. I was not going to be one of them.

I followed the program. I did lose some hair due to the yew tablets, I think. I started wearing wigs and liked them better than my own hair and I didn't have to fuss with my own hair, either. Besides, when I'm off the program, I fully expect my hair to come back.

There were tiny sores that came out on my skin, which I was told would happen. These were toxins coming out. I was not to lift anything heavy. The tonic softens muscles and tissues so that the cancer can pull out and be discarded. Other than that, there were no side effects.

About a month into the program, I started to feel pinching in the breast, and asked my friend about it, since she had gone through this. She said that she had pinching throughout her body. The cancer was breaking loose. One day, the pinching was so bad, I was wincing. She told me that was the core breaking free. I never felt another pain in the breast, even to this day.

Five months after I started on the Hoxsey program, I went back to the surgeon, who insisted I be rechecked. I was curious myself. Another mammogram was taken. She came into the room and gave me the results. "Well, I see the two scars from the double biopsy, but there's no evidence of cancer." She still wanted to remove the breast, however. No way, I told her. She insisted that she left margins in when she did the biopsy and was afraid it would come back. That was seven years ago.

I received letters from the radiologist and surgeon, letting me know that I was putting my health at risk and should return for treatment. It took a lot of courage and confidence for me to know what I was doing was right. Even my sister and mother let me know that they were worried— until they found out that the doctor could no longer see any cancer. It took a lot of strength to buck the system and those you love, and watch them worry about you. I was a salmon swimming upstream.

I then had my dosage of tonic cut back after four years. The program is a five-year program. In my last year, I was weaned off the tonic and yew tablets. By December 2005, I completed my five years and was off the treatment. If it ever should return, I will be given tonic free to me for the rest of my life. That is how confident they are that it works. They have a 70-80% success rate. The 20-30% failure is mostly due to people coming as a last resort (after chemo, radiation and surgery didn't work) or not following the diet and program. I was cautioned to stick as close to the diet as possible, as it is a healthier way to live anyway. That is no problem for me. In fact, I feel much better. I used to get headaches before the treatment, and since I changed my diet I hardly ever get headaches anymore.

So I had the choice of cutting, nuking and poisoning, including killing off my good cells, or building up my immune system and destroying the cancer naturally. I could submit to the medical treatments which save very few lives as compared with those who die from this dreaded disease under those treatments, or use natural and non-invasive methods to help my body fight the cancer itself. Which would you choose?

CASE SEVEN: PANCREATIC CANCER
BY LONA BURKHART

I am a long-time rancher, and I love it. I live by myself now with all of my animals, up here in Oregon on a roughly 5,000 acre ranch, off of the main gravel road, about fifty miles from the town of Madras. I raise quarter horses, and paints, and cattle. Back in 2004 I wasn't feeling good. I was getting older though, and expected to slow down a bit. I got to the point where I would get up in the morning and go feed the animals and then just come back inside and sleep. A good friend of mine, Rachel Hill, came to look at some of my horses. She is a very good friend, like a daughter to me. We were talking. She told me that I looked terrible, all yellow. Even my eyes looked yellow. She said that I needed to go to the doctor. So we arranged it. My doctor, Dr. Valenti, who I think walks on water, thought that I might have a liver problem, or that there might be an issue with the water which I get from a shallow well here at the ranch. It was expensive, but I had the water checked. It was fine. Still, I was getting sicker. Dr. Valenti did blood tests and an ultrasound. Even I could see the lump or mass on the ultrasound. It was a pretty good size. I was admitted to St. Charles Hospital, up in Bend, in central Oregon. It is a very good hospital. Those days are a bit hazy to me now, but they did tests, including something called a brush and two biopsies. Dr. Boone, the head oncologist, informed me that I had an advanced pancreatic cancer which had spread to the liver and lymph system. He said that, at that point, unfortunately, it was inoperable. He told me that there was nothing he could do, other than to control my pain. I told him that I was elderly, and not afraid to die. I had previously experienced what is known as a near-death experience. It confirmed to me that death was not to be feared. But I told him that I had many animals which needed my care, and that I needed to make arrangements for them, and could he give me his best estimate of how long I had. I had a friend who in the previous year had died from pancreatic cancer within thirty days of diagnosis. The estimate he gave me was also thirty days.

My granddaughter, Miranda Bosnan, and her husband live in southern California. I am extremely close to them. They came to stay with me at the ranch along with Rachel. In fact, you can't believe all of the good friends who started arriving and even camping outside, just to help me get my many animals and ranch affairs put in order. It was a sight to see! They brought their horses to round up my cattle, and equipment to shoe my horses, and on and on. Family and friends from Texas to Oregon held prayer sessions for me. I was very blessed. At one point there were thirty wonderful people here. In effect they were helping me to get ready to die. I felt guilty that I did not die after all! But at that time I was mostly trying to take care of my animals, giving away my pets, and giving away personal possessions that had been in the family for a lifetime.

Most of us ranchers who live outdoors in the sun get skin cancers. I had gotten some during the time that I lived in Fallon, Nevada. Someone had given me an external lotion they called cowboy mud. It is a black ointment related to what some call Indian mud. *(Editor's Note: Indian mud generally uses bloodroot as an active ingredient similar to the Hoxsey external cancer treatment)* There was an outfit in Reno that was selling it, and it darn sure did get rid of the skin cancer. There was a good friend of mine from those days who always suggested to me that I take a little bit of that cowboy mud, about the size of a pea, roll it up in some bread, and swallow it. She suggested that I should do so every month for prevention. But I had never done so. I just used the ointment on my face. But during this period my friend called and again suggested that I eat some of that medicine. My granddaughter started feeding me a little of the ointment in that manner, perhaps twice a day, for ten days or so. I am absolutely convinced that this is the reason that I was able to buy some time and not be in pain. It was taking extra time to round up all of the cattle, as the terrain can be difficult here. And during that same time, some of my friends were discussing relatives who had had good results treating cancer at the clinics down in Tijuana. There are many clinics there, but my friend Penny gave me the number for one of them, the Bio-Medical center. After my granddaughter contacted them, she advised me to get all of my medical records and to take the first flight to San Diego.

I contacted Dr. Valenti, who over many years had become a good family friend, even visiting my ranch with his family. When my biopsy had originally been taken, which turned out to be pancreatic cancer, he had been very kind to me and my granddaughter. At that time he had prayed with us for a miracle of healing. I explained that while he would probably not approve of my plan to go to Tijuana, that I felt I had nothing to lose, and that I would like to get a copy of my records and biopsy from him. He of course had them ready for me. I stopped by his office on the way to the airport in Redmond, and then flew on to San Diego.

My granddaughter and I stayed in a motel in San Ysidro, which is very close to the Mexican border, just on the outskirts of San Diego. Early the next morning we drove to the border and parked. We walked across and got a Mexican taxi to take us to the clinic. You do not need a reservation at the clinic, but you are supposed to be there first thing in the morning. My granddaughter had the address, and the taxi driver said that he knew where it was. But his English was poor, and our Spanish was poor, and he really did not know at all. The drive all over Tijuana, up and down the hills, looking for the clinic, in that cab, was terrible. It was an old Pontiac without much in the way of brakes. When the driver saw a stop signal it meant to him to try to beat everyone else through the intersection. We eventually found the clinic. I was exhausted. I did not know at that time that there is a much easier way. There is a shuttle every morning from the Best Western Americana motel in San Ysidro which will take you directly to the clinic and return you the same afternoon. But we made it that first time.

The people at the clinic are the nicest people. When you arrive, they take your records and give you a urine test and blood test, and take an x-ray. Then you wait in a comfortable room with the other patients for your turn to consult with the doctors. The building and the view are beautiful, up on the side of a hill. When our turn came, Miranda and I went in to speak with the doctor. He lay the blood tests which they had just done down next to the tests which I had brought from my Oregon hospital. There were actually many more markers checked on the Bio-Medical test than on my hospital test. The doctor said that it showed some slight stabilization already. I completely attribute that to the cowboy mud which I had been eating. The doctors at Bio-Medical do not hurry you. Miranda had a lot of questions for them. We then waited a little more, and were called back in for a physical exam. They carefully explained the various medicines and supplements, what they were for, and how to use them at home. If you look at the ingredients, there are some that you have probably never heard of, but some I think that are the same as in that cowboy mud. Of course the Hoxsey tonic has more ingredients and is very refined. It has a long history of success. But I don't think I would have even lived to get to the clinic if I hadn't eaten some of that mud. Then you leave. Of course we still had to deal with the taxi and the border that time. I can't stress enough how much easier it is to just take the shuttle in the first place.

I went back three more times for regular check ups at various intervals to the Bio-Medical Center in Tijuana. The last time I even brought another patient with me who was in a wheelchair. My own doctors here in Oregon gave me lots of blood tests and CAT scans. They just couldn't believe that the cancer was getting smaller and smaller. I did ultrasounds too. Then it was gone! My doctor here said that it was one of the two true miracles that he had seen in his life. Just as it is said that there are no atheists in a foxhole, I believe that there are also none with cancer. To me, prayer was very important, as was the kind doctors and staff of the Bio-Medical Center who worked to heal me. That was all eight years ago, and I am now eighty-one years old. I believe in standing up for what you know is right, and telling the truth about it. That is why I am not shy about telling my story. My phone number and address are available for people to talk with me through the Cancer Control Society in southern California. There have been many things in my life that might have been the end of me by now. I do not know what God has planned for me, but maybe he just wants me to help some folks yet before I go, so I am doing my best. That is my story.

CASE EIGHT: PANCREATIC CANCER/PANCREATITIS
BY CAROL MAIN

My name is Carol. My husband and I moved to Alaska in 1983. It wasn't long before I was sick. Finally I went to the local doctor and he ran some tests, including an ultrasound.

The local doctor was nice but knew I was in serious trouble. My problem was the pancreas. He said he didn't want to touch me, so he said he wanted to send me to Anchorage. The one he wanted to send me to was gone right then, but he didn't want me to wait, so he sent me to another "specialist".

I asked this doctor how long I had to live. He scrunched his face up, rolled his eyes around as he looked around at the ceiling and said, "Maaaybe, just maybe, six months." The way he said it, I knew he felt there was no way I would live anywhere near that much longer. I also knew it, I was so sick that if I had lived two months more, I would have really been surprised.

I left his office with a death sentence, no hope for anything, I felt like I had a shovel on my shoulder. I was not afraid to die, I know what the Bible really teaches about death and so I don't really fear it, But, I had two sons who were four and six years old at the time. We had moved from California to Alaska solely for the purpose of home-schooling them. I loved my boys and husband so much and wanted desperately to see the boys grow up safe and sound. It all looked so hopeless at that point.

The stress of all this worrying about my husband and sons, etcetera, really took its toll on me. My mind shut down where I could hardly think at all. I couldn't hold a conversation. By the time someone finished a sentence, I didn't have any idea of even the subject they were talking about, let alone what they were saying about it. I was a complete mess.

Soon after, my husband Bernie told a friend at work how sick I was. The friend told my husband to call Jill. Jill had gone to the Hoxsey Bio-Medical Center years before and had good results. I called Jill and she really encouraged me to call Mildred, the lady who ran the clinic at the time. I kept telling Jill that I had no money and Mildred wouldn't care. She kept insisting I call anyway and so I finally did. I still remember explaining my situation to Mildred and when she heard pancreas, she said in a very rough, matter of fact voice, "GET DOWN HERE

{*thistle flower*}

IMMEDIATELY!" I said, "Lady, I have no money, I could barely scrape together a plane ticket." She said, "Well, the important thing is to get you well! You can worry about that some other time!!!" I was completely shocked; here was someone who actually cared! She really cared more about me than she cared about money!

By the time I talked to Mildred, I was so sick I could barely stand up. I knew she was my only hope. I had never been to Tijuana, Mexico and I had no idea what their treatment was like, but at that time I didn't care. I knew it was do or die, so within a few days I was headed to the little airport in Kenai, Alaska. Bernie and I couldn't afford a ticket for him too, so I had to go alone.

I discovered it was not scary a bit to go to Tijuana to the clinic. I only had to go for one day. I met Mildred and found her to be very nice and genuinely concerned. At the end of the day, she told me what to do and said to come back in 6 months! I was not given an automatic death sentence! There was some hope! I about fell over.

I had been treated very kindly at the clinic, with dignity, patience, and understanding. They talked to me like I did have a brain and my body was my business. They explained everything to me like I was an intelligent person. They explained that I had either very severe pancreatitis or pancreatic cancer. Mildred also agreed that at that time there was no test to know for sure, but she said if it wasn't cancer yet, it was just ready to be. So she said, "We'll treat is like it is!" They didn't want me to be cut on and have it spread just to name it exactly, she wanted me to get well. She knew I was in deep trouble, but she didn't panic, she just told me what to do and said to come back. Now it was up to me.

When Mildred told me to come back, it was a real turning point for me. My mind started clearing up right away. I had something to look forward to. I was told not to cheat on the eating program at all. The doctor also really stressed this to me so I didn't. I read every label, I did not eat in restaurants and take chances like that, and I never ate food someone else prepared. I knew exactly what I was eating all the time. With the Hoxsey program, you have to be careful to avoid certain foods, because they ruin the herbal tonic they give you. If you ruin the tonic, then it simply won't work. I have watched for many years now and have seen many people stick to the eating program like they should and I've watched many who didn't. The results are unquestionably different. It's totally ridiculous to think any doctor or any clinic will have 100% success treating every kind of cancer in everyone all the time, but for those who are willing to follow the diet and treatment exactly as they should, the results are often tremendous.

The Hoxsey Clinic, (Bio-Medical Center) also cured my husband when he had lymphoma. He had a large tumor in his chest and some in his neck. He was unable to talk for six-and-a-half months. No one in our town ever thought he would talk again, except me. I already knew how good the clinic was and when my husband decided to go there, I was completely put at ease. He was the type to stick to a program and he did. His voice eventually returned and the tumors completely disappeared and never returned. He really made believers out of a lot of people.

I will always be very appreciative to the clinic, and to Mildred. Over the years I grew to love Mildred very much and will always remember her as being one of the most caring people I have ever known. I also have grown to love the doctor who has worked there for well over 20 years and the staff who have also worked for many years along side him tirelessly giving of themselves to help others. Now Liz, Mildred's sister, is doing an excellent job of running the clinic and I also find her to be very kind and caring, so, she too has found her way into my heart. I can only say, "Thank you so very much to each and every one of them."

Editor's Note: Following her recovery, Carol Main, at considerable time and personal expense, produced an excellent video documentary showing the Bio-Medical Center's everyday operations and interviewing many patients for their personal stories. It is entitled, **The Experience** *and is available both through the Bio-Medical Center, or by contacting Carol through email at carolmain@yahoo.com (put "Hoxsey" or "Bio-Medical" in the subject to avoid accidental deletion). Carol has stated that she is happy to be of assistance and council to others with questions involving the Hoxsey treatment at the Bio-Medical Center.)*

CASE NINE: BREAST CANCER
BY MARION KINCAID

Cancer. The very word conjures up a myriad of emotions. Fear being the primary one. Denial. Uncertainty. Death.

All these loom larger in the mind. Fortunately, we are spirit as well as mind and body—spirit speaks to us whether we are listening or not. Choose to listen.

I was the last person one would select as "most likely to choose a naturopathy therapy in response to a cancer diagnosis." I had worked in what I refer to as the edge of allopathic medicine—a receptionist for a large multi-national pharmaceutical company; the assistant to nurses and a dietician in the "wellness" program of a major hospital; the assistant to even more nurses in a big toxic-chemical court case involving 2,000 claimants; and recently, quality assurance specialist in another big hospital/pharmaceutical supply company.

Thus when my first diagnosis of breast cancer came, I started out on the allopathic path. I did the biopsy, the next surgery (at that time, a segmectomy and a lymph-node check). Nothing was detected in the lymph-nodes; the surgeon had, he thought, all the cancer out and clear margins. Still, he was recommending radiation, and five years of tamoxifen. So I proceeded to arrange for the radiation treatment. Everything was on schedule—except the day came and I didn't go to the radiation center. The decision not to go, I think, was made during a process I had started; one that I turn to when I am in trouble.

And so, I started praying—*what on earth should I do now, Lord?* I wanted to get well. From this a series of events occurred… while looking in the trash can for something to read on the subway home from work, I pulled out an alternative newspaper that had on the last page a whole page ad for the A.R.E. (Association for Research and Enlightenment). I had heard of the A.R.E., Cayce and his work; however, I did not know there was a conference center, 800 number and so forth.

This was the turning point. It led me to counsel with Dr. Bill McGarey in Arizona over the phone. He outlined for me a process to use in how to safely venture inward. I was first to meditate for fifteen minutes before going to sleep… to get a question really clear in my mind. When I asked what kind of question, he suggested, "Why don't you ask if you are sick?" Then I was to go to sleep and when I woke up, note "the answer." It did not seem a difficult process. And so I did so for about a week.

Cayce says when there is a need, the answers will be there. Was I sick? Just as I was about to come to full consciousness, I was telling my girlfriend from Milwaukee to stop sending the "get well" cards. Thus, not sick any longer! Should I pursue chemotherapy? A big *"no"*! And so, I only took two months of tamoxifen. How should I handle the nurses at work who were getting increasingly uneasy? The dream—I was playing in a quartet with three others playing the strings, and I, the drums. I was beating to my own drum—*(beating my own drum or marching to my own drumbeat??).* Later, I was to learn this was called "incubating a dream."

Since I was only four hours from the A.R.E. in the Washington, D.C. area, I started coming to conferences, meeting people, reading from the library, and finding like-minded groups in the D.C. area. All of this was immersing me more into Cayce, alternative medicine, new ideas and eventually new ways.

A year later, the second diagnosis came, a lump in the other breast. This time, the surgeon asked me what I wanted to do. I told him I wanted to go to a "Holistic" clinic in Phoenix. I went through the "Temple Beautiful" eleven day residential program at Bill McGarey's A.R.E. clinic in Phoenix. By the end of the program, I had a pretty clear idea of what to do; however, incorporating the program in a routine with working full-time was difficult. After attempting to do so for six months, I told the surgeon, if the tumor is still here, schedule me for surgery. It was still there.

Another segmectomy (no lymph-node check this time)… and after the surgery, the doctor said, "Well this (indicator) is favorable, this is favorable, this is favorable…" He went through his whole list of indications for a good (or not so good) prognosis. And, "You are probably correct that there is no lymph-node activity." I just said, "Thank you, Doctor." And mentally, "Thank you, God!" The visualization techniques that I learned at the A.R.E clinic, I feel, had stopped any lymph-node activity. Two more months of tamoxifen followed.

In 1996, I moved to Virginia Beach and resumed life. I am grateful for all those years of living what a "normal" life consists of—even if mundane at times.

With the year 2005 came the third diagnosis of breast cancer. I thought, "I know the routine." Not exactly! This time, it was a different surgeon in a different city. And this time, I did suspect it had not only returned, but since my arms were in pain, that lymph-node involvement was there. I did not suspect what the surgeon would suggest after the biopsy (again confirming the cancer diagnosis); he suggested two variations of a mastectomy. After getting a second opinion...which merely confirmed the first scenario, I came to see this as a choice which is "S.O.P.", standard operating procedure in the medical world. I viewed this as virtually a no-win choice. Surely, there must be another way.

And so, I was praying again. Eventually, over the next two months, I went to three different doctors of osteopathy in the area, with various suggestions on what to do. One of the doctors recommended a book called *The Complete Cancer Cleanse: A Proven Program to Detoxify and Renew Body, Mind, and Spirit* by Cherie Calbom, M.S., John Calbom, M.A., and Michael Mahaffey, P.C. Mahaffey is a cancer survivor of over twenty years! While looking for this book I called up the A.R.E. library and was greeted and assisted in my search by the librarian.

That very afternoon I went to the library and picked up a wealth of information on Cayce and cancer, herbal treatment, and the Bio-Medical Center located in Tijuana, Mexico. Roger Bloom's small book entitled *Cancer Medicine From Nature: The Herbal Cancer Formulas of Edgar Cayce and Harry Hoxsey,* was the most informative. Bloom, an A.R.E. member, had investigated Cayce's herbal formulas when his parents had diagnoses of cancer. He provided a thorough comparison of Cayce's herbal formulas and Harry Hoxsey's formulas used at the Bio-Medical Center in Mexico.

Roger Bloom's presentation of Cayce and Hoxsey, and my own desire to avoid the "choice" of more surgery/radiation/chemotherapy, had coalesced into my reevaluation of herbal medicine. Now, instead of thinking herbal medicine was "backward" or "ineffectual," I saw it as a return to the early days of the pharmaceutical industry. I saw herbs as closer to nature and therefore more effective (and with fewer side effects).

The librarian also put me in touch with others in the A.R.E. community who have started the Hoxsey treatment from the Bio-Medical Center. All are veterans... three-and-a-half years into the five year program. I was able to reach one woman who also had had breast cancer. She was very helpful in answering all of my questions.

The way opened for me and a friend to go to the Bio-Medical Center a little over two weeks after receiving the library materials. Set upon a hill in Tijuana,

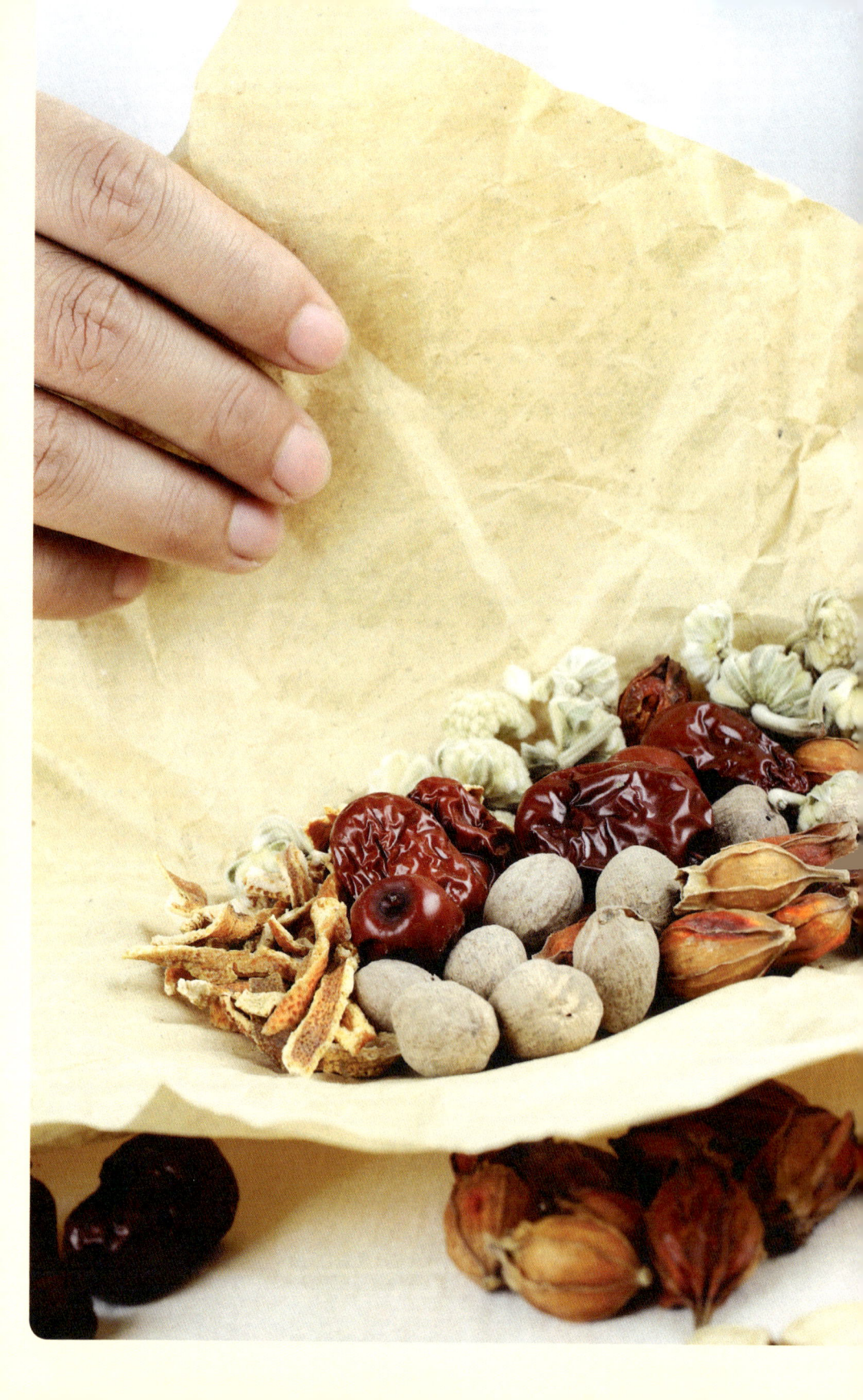

with a view that just glimpses the Pacific Ocean, and with a grand balcony adjacent to the main waiting room, hope was in the air. Patients are chatting among themselves. A video was shown on how to prepare "the tonic" and about the dietary guidelines that accompany the program. Sprinkled alongside the practical information are comments from real people who have recovered from their cancers. You see yourself mirrored among these faces, and hope for you begins to dawn and grow.

The herbs and diet recommendations are all to support your body in becoming and maintaining an alkaline state. Exactly what Cayce recommends! Thus, no pork, vinegar, tomatoes, or alcohol. Stay away from white flour, sugar. Watch the salt! The surprise was "no microwave." My kitchen is being reordered.

In fact, my life is being reordered. I have started once again to ask myself, "Well if I am still here, what else, Lord, can I do?" And as always, answers are coming. Change is in the air as this new year of 2007 has begun.

And the cancer? I have been on the herbal treatment for a year. After about three months, the pain in my arms had gone! My yearly checkup included both mammograms and a pap test. Both were *"normal."* Thank God for people like Cayce, Hoxsey, Bloom, folks at the A.R.E. and the A.R.E. community, and some very wonderful angels. God Bless you all!

Endnotes

1. FitzGerald, Benedict. *A Report by Special Council for a US Senate Investigating Committee Making a Fact-Finding Study of a Conspiracy Against the Health of the American People,* Congressional Record, Vol. 99, Part 12, pp 4045-52, 83rd Congress, 1st session, 7.2.53-8.28.53.

2. Hoxsey, Harry M. 1956. You Don't Have to Die. New York: Milestone Books.

3. Ausubel, Kenny. 2000. When Healing Becomes A Crime, The Amazing Story of the Hoxsey Cancer Clinics and the Return of Alternative Therapies, Rochester, VT: Healing Arts Press.

4. Kirkpatrick, Sidney D. 2000. Edgar Cayce, An American Prophet. New York: Riverhead Books (Penquin Putnam).

5. The Edgar Cayce Foundation. 1995. The Complete Edgar Cayce Readings on CD-ROM. Virginia Beach, VA: A.R.E. Press; URL: www.edgarcayce. org.

6. Walters, Richard. OPTIONS, The Alternative Cancer Therapy Book, Avery, Garden City Park, New York, 1993.

7. Sattilaro, Anthony J. with Monte, Tom. 1982. Recalled By Life, The Story of My Recovery From Cancer. Houghton Mifflin, Boston.

8. Winters, Sir Jason. 1990. The Jason Winters Story. Las Vegas, NV: Vinton.

9. Wigmore, Ann, 1985. The Wheatgrass Book, Wayne, N.J.: Avery.

10. Thomas, Richard. 1993. The Essiac Report, Canada's Remarkable Unknown Cancer Remedy. Los Angeles: Alternative Treatment Information Network.

11. Brown, Tom Jr. 1985. Tom Brown's Guide to Wild Edible and Medicinal Plants. New York: Berkley.

12. Shufer, Vickie, Editor, "The Wild Foods Forum," Virginia Beach, VA: Eco Images

13. Duke, James A. 1997. The Green Pharmacy, Emmaus, PA: Rodale Press, 1997.

14. Hoxsey, Harry M. (see Footnote 2)

15. Ibid.

16. Hartwell, Jonathan L. 1982. Plants Used Against Cancer, Lawrence, MA: Quartermain.

17. Ausubel, Kenny. (see Footnote 3)

18. Kloss, Jethro. 1971. Back To Eden, New York: Beneficial Books.

19. Ausubel, Kenny. (see Footnote 3)

20. The Edgar Cayce Foundation. (see Footnote 5)

21. Ibid.

22. The Cayce Herbal. URL: www.meridianinstitute.com.

23. Informational Pamplet, BIO-MEDICAL CENTER, Hoxsey Therapy Offering Hope and Recovery. Tijuana, Baja California, Mexico: Bio- Medical Ctr., 2001. 24.

24. Thomas, Richard. (see Footnote 10)

25. Ward, Patricia Spain. "History Of The Hoxsey Treatment Contract Report to the Office of Technology Assessment 1987." Reprinted in Townsend Letter for Doctors and Patients. 5.97.

26. Duke, James A. Personal Correspondence.

27. The Cayce Herbal. (see Footnote 22)

28. The Edgar Cayce Foundation. (see Footnote 5)

29. Uckun et al, "Pokeweed antiviral protein as a potent inhibitor of human immunodeficiency virus," Antimicrobial Agents and Chemotherapy. Vol 42, No. 2, 1998, pp. 383-388.

30. The Edgar Cayce Foundation. (see Footnote 5)

31. Ibid.

32. Ausubel, Kenny. (see Footnote 3)

33. Jones, Eli. 1911. Cancer: Its Causes, symptoms, and Treatment. Boston: Therapeutic.

34. Ralph W. Moss. 1998. Herbs Against Cancer. Brooklyn NY: Equinox.

35. Duke, James A. Personal Correspondence.

36. Ward, Patricia Spain. (see Footnote 25)

37. The Cayce Herbal. (see Footnote 22)

38. The Edgar Cayce Foundation. (see Footnote 5)

39. Ausubel, Kenny. (see Footnote 3)

40. Hartwell, Jonathan L. (see Footnote 16)

41. Duke, James A. Personal Correspondence.

42. Ibid.

43. The Edgar Cayce Foundation. (see Footnote 5)

44. Ibid.

45. Ibid.

46. Ibid.

47. The Cayce Herbal. (see Footnote 22)

48. Ward, Patricia Spain. (see Footnote 25)

49. Hartwell, Jonathan L. (see Footnote 16)

50. Ausubel, Kenny. (see Footnote 3)

51. The Cayce Herbal. (see Footnote 22)

52. The Edgar Cayce Foundation. (see Footnote 5)

53. Ibid.

54. Ibid.

55. Ausubel, Kenny. (see Footnote 3)

56. Ibid.
57. The Cayce Herbal. (see Footnote 22)
58. The Edgar Cayce Foundation. (see Footnote 5)
59. The Cayce Herbal. (see Footnote 22)
60. Ausubel, Kenny. (see Footnote 3)
61. Hartwell, Jonathan L. (see Footnote 16)
62. Duke, James A. Personal Correspondence.
63. Ausubel, Kenny. (see Footnote 3)
64. Ibid.
65. The Cayce Herbal. (see Footnote 22)
66. The Edgar Cayce Foundation. (see Footnote 5)
67. Ibid.

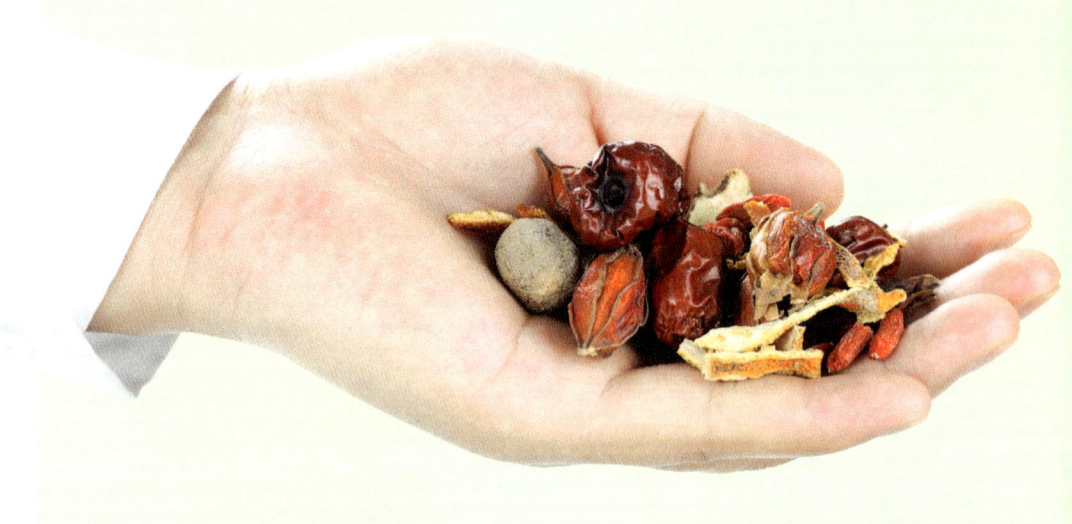

Appendix A: Examples of Simple Plant Preparations

Select Listing of Important Healing Plants

Perhaps the easiest way to take advantage of healing plants is to make teas with them, or simply eat them cooked or raw. Companies also specialize in making fluid extracts and tinctures of healing plants which can be added to water or juice. Such extracts are available in health food stores, online, and available from companies listed in the resource section of this book. Here is a very short and simple list of some of the more important plants that are healing in cases of cancer, and how to use them. The medicinal properties of most of these are covered in detail in the text or may be found in the books listed as resources.

RED CLOVER BLOSSOMS (TRIFOLIUM PRETENSE)
Red clover blossoms can be picked and eaten raw, added to salads raw, or steeped to make tea.

BURDOCK ROOT (ARCTIUM LAPPA)
Burdock root is eaten raw in salads by the Japanese where it is called Gobo. It can be found in specialty food stores fresh or dug in the wild. It is a sweet, crispy, moist addition to salads. Burdock root is also available in most health food stores as a tea.

DANDELION ROOT (TARAXACUM OFFICIANALE)
Dandelion is of course well known as a weed to the average gardener. Its leaves are becoming more well known as ingredients of fresh salads in trendy restaurants. Some day it will be more appreciated as the powerful cleansing medicine that it is. Dandelion may be eaten fresh, or sautéed to remove bitterness. The roots when baked and powdered are a common coffee substitute. Dandelion tea and occasionally coffee is available in markets. The entire plant is edible.

YELLOW DOCK ROOT (RUMEX CRISPUS)
Yellow dock root is most often found in health stores as a tea. It is a very common plant found in open grassy fields, like the dandelion. Its leaves may be eaten raw or cooked.

POKE ROOT (PHYTOLACCA AMERICANA)
Poke has some of the most powerful anti-cancer effects of any. Medicine. It cannot be safely eaten raw. The root is used in very small quantity in medicines. The leaves of young plants may be eaten just

like any other cooked green if twice boiled briefly and the water thrown away. The juice of fresh poke leaves, when mixed with Vaseline, was available commercially in the past and used extensively by Dr. Eli Jones to treat skin cancers. I have easily made this salve at home from the description in Dr. Jones' book and found it successful. Poke is not only powerful, it is also plentiful. Once identified with certainty, it can be prepared following the information in the Edgar Cayce readings, or the formulas left by Dr. Eli Jones. Several of Dr. Jones' most important herbal formulas have been reproduced and are available from Ingrid Naiman's website, *cancersalves.com*. This site provides a great service to cancer patients, and the products are reasonably priced. Still, it is important to remember that the great healing power of the poke plant is available just outside in nature and is free to all.

GOLDENSEAL (HYDRASTUS CANADENSIS)
Goldenseal root is not as easily found as the previous plants but is commonly available in health food stores either as a bulk powder or in tea bags. It is simple to consume as tea. Because the taste is bitter, it is often combined with other teas such as licorice or mint to make it more palatable. Goldenseal root was used by native Americans to heal cancer. It is also internally healing to mucous membranes. Goldenseal and myrrh are often used together to both disinfect and heal even serious external wounds and infections.

COMMON PLANTAIN (PLANTAGO MAJOR)
Plantain is a short broad leaved plant found in lawns and at the edge of fields. It is one of the most common and available of species and also the most useful. (A different plant with banana-like fruits has the same common name). Its leaves can be crushed and applied directly to bites and wounds. They help draw out poisons and infection. Plantain seeds can be easily harvested and eaten to provide considerable protein and fiber. A tea of plantain can remove intestinal parasites. Edgar Cayce gave instructions for preparing an external healing salve for use in cases of skin cancer using a combination of plantain and cream.

PINE (PINUS)
All types of pine trees have evergreen needles, which when steeped in hot water make a delicious tea that is extremely high in vitamin C. Also, the very thin soft inner bark is very high in protein and was dried and made into bread by native Americans Removal of outer bark can be tedious; however the needles are very convenient to gather.

References

Formulae

More sophisticated herbal combinations can be formulated at home, following the methods found in the Edgar Cayce readings. Often, Cayce would specify that a few ounces of various fresh or dried herbs be added to a gallon of rainwater in a non-aluminum pot. Then the mixture should be simmered, not boiled, until about one-fourth of the original liquid remains. This is strained to remove the fibrous material and usually a few ounces of grain alcohol (100% alcohol), with a little balsam of tolu, would be added as preservative. The dosage would usually be between one and three teaspoons, four times daily; thirty minutes before meals and at bedtime. This is simple enough that almost anyone can undertake it.

The following is an actual formula inspired by both the Cayce and Hoxsey formulas, which I have made at home and used personally. It is important not to exceed the amount of mandrake root in this formula, as it is a powerful liver regulator, and is very carefully limited in the Cayce readings. Do not experiment unless you are working under professional guidance. Also, stop and seek professional advice if you are nursing, pregnant or may become pregnant.

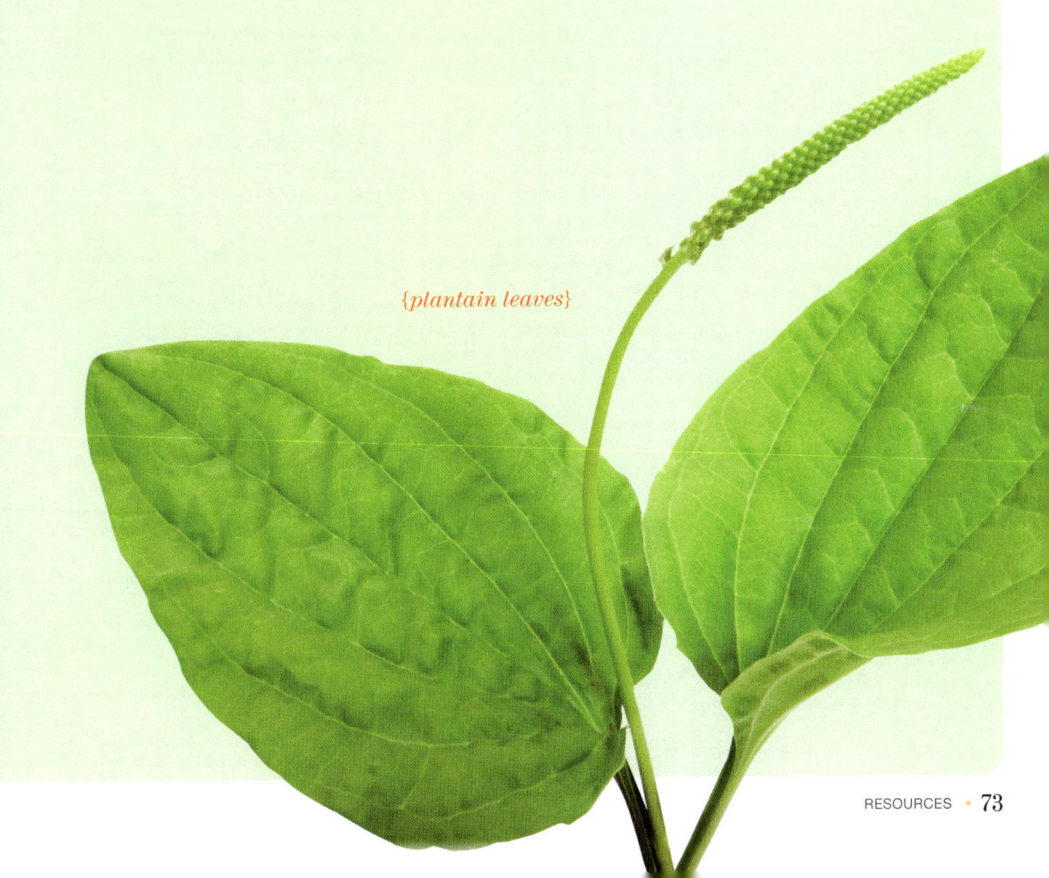

{plantain leaves}

CAYCE/HOXSEY INSPIRED HERBAL FORMULA

To one gallon of rain or distilled water add:

sarsaparilla root (Smilax officinalis) .... 2 ounces
wild cherry bark (Prunus serotina)................... 2 ounces
burdock root (Arctium lappa)........................... 2 ounces
yellow dock root (Rumex crispus) .... 2 ounces
poke root, dried (Phytolacca americana)......... ¾ ounce
prickley ash bark (Zanthoxylum americanum).. 1 ounce
red clover blossoms (Trifolium pretense)........ 2 ounces
stillingia root (Stillingia sylvatica)..................... ½ ounce
goldenseal (Hydrastus canadensis).................. ¾ ounce
mandrake root (Podophyllum peltatum).......... 20 grains
        (480 grains = one ounce is the conversion)
buchu leaves (Barasoma ovata)....................... 30 grains
elder blossoms (Sambuchus canadensis) ...... 4 ounces
sassafras root bark (Sassafras albidum) .... 1 ounce
calisaya bark (Cinchona calisaya)..................... 1 ounce

Simmer these herbs until only a quarter of the original water is left, or about one quart or one liter. Then strain out the plants from the liquid. To the remaining liquid add the following:

grain alcohol .... 4 ounces
with 3 drams of balsam tolu (Myroxylon balsamum) shaved in
        (4 drams = one fluid ounce is the conversion)

While using this formula, potassium iodide (KI) was also taken as a supplement. The dosage was approximately 130 mg per day, which is a commonly available over-the-counter dosage.

A member of my family used this formula for an extended period, and felt that it provided health benefits, as well as having an enjoyable taste. The above formula is a personal example only, and need not have this many ingredients in order to be helpful. If we believe the experience of Edgar Cayce, Jethro Kloss, Dr. Eli Jones and many others, a formula prepared from even a few of these ingredients, those most easily recognized and gathered around one's own home, prepared in a similar manner, should have great healing potential.

References

Formulas from Dr. Eli Jones, M.D.

Dr. Jones was an American doctor at the turn of the twentieth century licensed in allopathic medicine, eclectic medicine and homeopathic medicine. He wrote the textbook *Cancer, Its Causes, Symptoms, and Treatment: Giving the Results of Over Forty Years' Experience in the Medical Treatment of this Disease.*

CERATE PHYTOLACCA FOLIUM (FOR EXTERNAL SKIN USE)

This ointment for early skin cancers is simple to make and reported by Jones in his text to be very effective.

20% juice of the leaves of poke (Phytolacca americana)
80% petroleum jelly (such as Vaseline)

COMPOUND SYRUP PHYTOLACCA

fluid extract of
  green poke root (Phytolacca americana) ...... 2 ounces
fluid extract of gentian (Gentiana lutea) .... ½ ounce
fluid extract of dandelion (Teraxacum officinale) 1 ounce

COMPOUND SYRUP SCROPHULARIA

figwort leaves & root (Scrophularia nodosa) 32 ounces
poke root (Phytolacca Americana) .... 8 ounces
yellow dock root (Rumex crispus) .... 8 ounces
American bittersweet (Celastrus scandens) ... 4 ounces
turkey corn root (Corydalis formosa) .... 2 ounces
American mandrake or
  mayapple root (Podophyllum peltatum) .... 4 ounces
juniper berries (Juniperus communis) .... 3 ounces
prickly ash berries (Zanthoxylum americanum) .. 1 ounce
guaiacum wood (Guaiacum officinale) .... 2 ounces

Dr. Jones specified a complex distillation procedure for this formula using alcohol in a steam displacement apparatus. A current day reproduction of this formula is available from www.sacredmedicinesanctuary.com.

Formula from Dr. John R. Christopher

Dr. Christopher was a renowned herbalist and founder of the School of Natural Healing.

ANTI-CANCER REMEDY

Equal parts:
red clover blossums (Trifolium praetense)
poke root (Phytolacca Americana)
licorice root (Glycyrrhiza glabra)
cascara sagrada (Rhamnus purshiana)
sarsaparilla root (Smilax officinalis)
prickly ash bark (Zanthoxylum americanum)
burdock root (Arctium lappa)
buckthorn bark (Rhamnus cathartica)
stillingia root (Stillingia sylvatica)
oregon grape root (Mahonia aquifolium)
peach bark (Prunus persica)
chaparral leaves (Larrea tridentate)

One teaspoon to one cup of boiling water, gradually working up to one cup, three times per day.

Jason Winters' Tea

red clover (Trifolium praetense)
chaparral (Larrea tridentate)
cayenne (Capsicum annuum)

(as listed in *Cancer Salves*, by Ingrid Naiman)

Renee Caisse's Essiac Tea

burdock (Arctium lappa)	52 parts
Indian rhubarb (Rheum officinale)	16 parts
sheep sorrel (Rumex acetosella)	1 part
slippery elm (Ulmus rubra)	4 parts
kelp (Laminaria)	2 parts
red clover (Trifolium praetense)	1 part
blessed thistle (Cnicus benedictus)	1 part
watercress (Nasturtium officinale)	4 parts

References

Bio-Medical Center Dry Herbal Capsule Ingredients

licorice (Glycrrhiza glabra)
red clover (Trifolium praetense)
burdock root (Arctium lappa)
European barberry (Berberis vulgaris)
cascara sagrada (Rhamnus purshiana)
prickly ash bark (Zanthoxylum americanum)
rhubarb (Rheum officinale)
chaparral (Larrea tridentate)
sarsaparilla (Smilax officinales)
turmeric (Curcuma longa)
pau d'arco (Tabebuia impetiginosa)

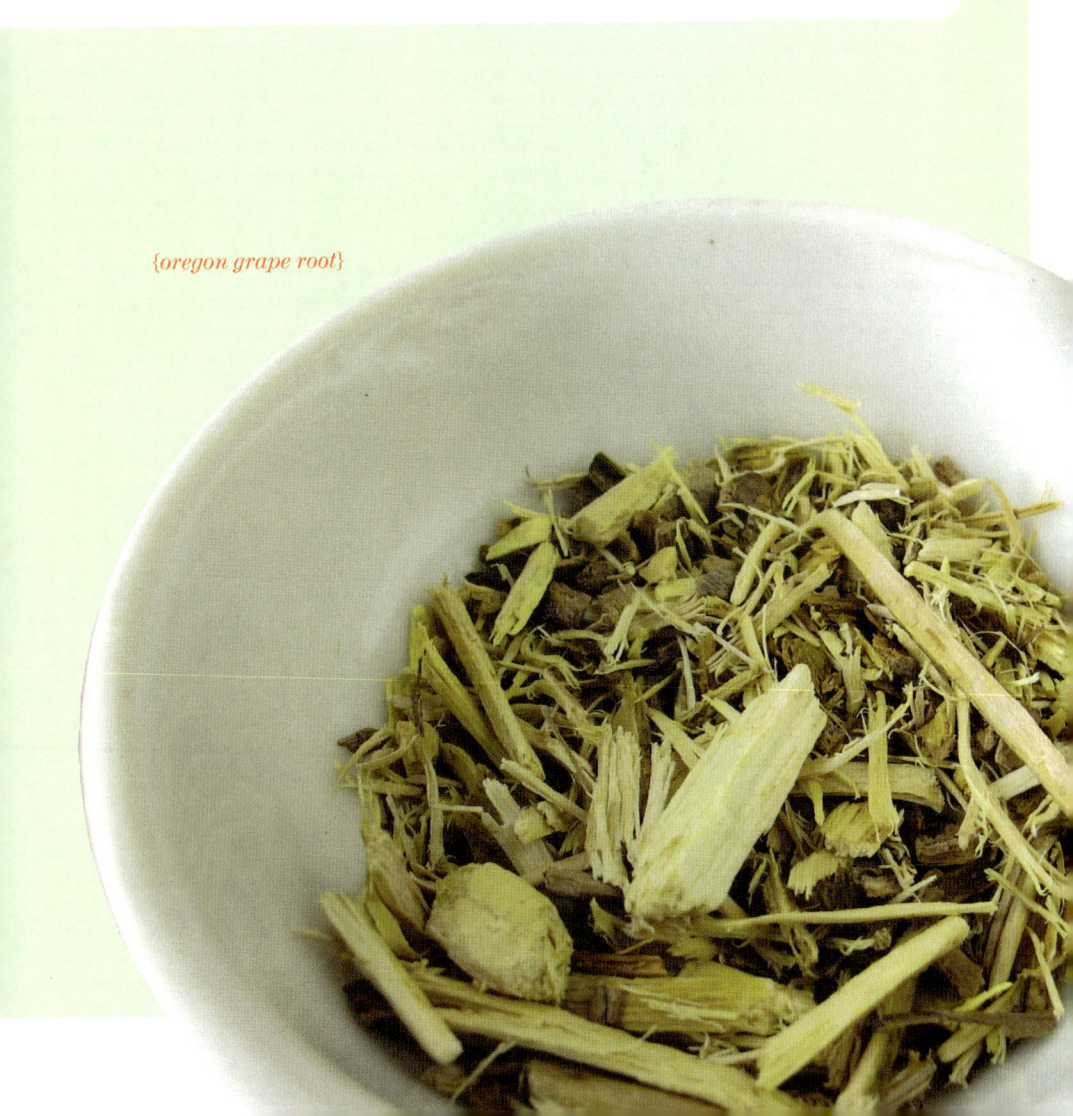

{oregon grape root}

Resources

Internet Resources

WWW.ANNWIGMORE.ORG
This is the website of Ann Wigmore, a lifelong advocate for the nutritional benefits of wheat grass juice, and the founder of the Hippocrates Institute.

WWW.BAAR.COM
This is the website of Baar products. Baar is the official manufacturer and distributor of health care products based upon the Edgar Cayce readings.

WWW.BEATING-CANCER-GENTLY.COM
This is the website of Bill Henderson, author of books, newsletters, and radio host, concerned with promoting simple, inexpensive and gentle alternative cancer therapies.

WWW.BREASTCANCERCHOICES.ORG
This is an informational website with extensive information on the role of iodine in cancer. It also hosts a very active and sophisticated email based user forum which is open to all.

WWW.CANCERCONTROLSOCIETY.COM
The Cancer Control Society is a non-profit organization which helps disseminate current information on alternative medical therapies. Its yearly symposium in Los Angeles draws distinguished medical speakers from around the world.

WWW.CANCERDECISIONS.COM
This is the website of Ralph Moss, Ph.D. Dr. Moss has, for decades, evaluated standard and alternative cancer treatments, written numerous books, films, newsletters and scientific articles on the subject, advised the National Institute of Health and provided personal advice and customized research for individuals.

WWW.EDGARCAYCE.ORG
This is the website of the non-profit Association for Research and Enlightenment. The organization was formed by Edgar Cayce in 1931 to promote the study of spirituality and holistic health.

WWW.GERSON.ORG
This is the website of the non-profit Gerson Institute, which educates patients and caregivers in administering the Gerson Therapy, an alternative non-toxic therapy for cancer and other degenerative

diseases. Max Gerson M.D. was described by Dr. Albert Schweitzer as "...one of the most imminent geniuses in the history of medicine".

WWW.HOLISTICCANCERSOLUTIONS.COM
This is the website of Eclectic Medicine International. This medical information service focuses on the latest research in non-toxic cancer treatments.

HTTP://LPI.OREGONSTATE.EDU
This is the website of the Linus Pauling Institute at Oregon State University. It is an excellent source of information concerning micronutrients, phytochemicals, supplements and health. Linus Pauling was the only two-time unshared winner of the Nobel Prize (Chemistry 1954, Peace 1962).

WWW.OUTSMARTYOURCANCER.COM
This is the website of author Tanya Pierce. Her book is an up-to-date review of the most successful alternative cancer therapies, including the Hoxsey Therapy.

WWW.SACREDMEDICINESANCTUARY.COM
This is one of the websites of Ingrid Naiman. Her company manufactures and distributes many rare ayurvedic and western herbal health products, including reproductions of the formulas of Eli Jones, M.D., and combinations similiar to those used by Harry Hoxsey.

Herbal Resources

MOUNTAIN ROSE HERBS
www.mountainroseherbs.com

P.O. Box 50220
Eugene, Oregon 97405 USA

(800)879-3337 or (541) 741-7307

RIDGE RUNNER TRADING COMPANY
199 Jefferson Road
Boone, North Carolina 28607 USA

(828) 264-3615

STARWEST BONTANICALS
www.starwest-botanicals.com

11253 Trade Center Drive
Rancho Cordova, California 95742 USA

(800) 800-4372 or (916) 638-8100

Recommended Reading

Ausubel, Kenny. ***When Healing Becomes a Crime: The Amazing Story of the Hoxsey Cancer Clinics and the Return of Alternative Therapies.*** Publisher: Healing Arts Press; 1st edition, May 1, 2000. ISBN-13: 978-0892819256

Boik, John. ***Cancer and Natural Medicine: A Textbook of Basic Science and Clinical Research.*** Publisher: Oregon Medical Press, 1995. ISBN-13: 0-964828006

Boik, John. ***Natural Compounds in Cancer Therapy: Promising Nontoxic Antitumor Agents from Plants and Other Natural Sources.*** Publisher: Oregon Medical Press; March 2001. ISBN-13: 0-964828014

Frahm, Anne E., with David J. Frahm. ***A Cancer Battle Plan: Six Strategies for Beating Cancer from a Recovered "Hopeless Case".*** Publisher: Tarcher; 1st edition, December 29, 1997. ISBN-13: 978-0874778939

Gerson, Charlotte, with Beata Bishop. ***Healing The Gerson Way: Defeating Cancer and Other Chronic Diseases.*** Publisher: Totality Books; 2nd edition, 2009. ISBN-13: 978-0976018629

Gerson, M.D., Max. ***A Cancer Therapy: Results of Fifty Cases and the Cure of Advanced Cancer by Diet Therapy: A Summary of 30 Years of Clinical Experimentation.*** Publisher: Station Hill Press; May 1997. ISBN-13: 978-0882682037

Issels, M.D., Josef. ***Cancer: A Second Opinion.*** Publisher: Square One Publishers; February 2005. ISBN-13: 978-0757002793

Jones, M.D., Eli G. ***Cancer, Its Causes, Symptoms and Treatment: Giving the Results of Over Forty Years' Experience in the Medical Treatment of This Disease.*** Publisher: Nabu Press; February 12, 2010. ISBN-13: 978-1144367501

Jochems, Ruth. ***Dr. Moerman's Anti-Cancer Diet: Holland's Revolutionary Nutritional Program for Combating Cancer.*** Publisher: Avery; January 1, 1995. ISBN-13: 978-0895294395

Kirkpatrick, Sydney D. ***Edgar Cayce, An American Prophet.*** Publisher: Penguin Group; 2000. ISBN-13: 978-1573228961

Kloss, Jethro. ***Back to Eden.*** Publisher: Back to Eden Publishing; January 22, 2004. ISBN-13: 978-0940985094

McMakin, Carolyn. ***Frequency Specific Microcurrent in Pain Management.*** Publisher: Churchill Livingstone; December 21, 2010. ISBN-13: 978-0443069765

Moss, Ph.D., Ralph W. *The Cancer Industry*. Publisher: Equinox Press; October 8, 1996. ISBN-13: 978-1881025092

Naiman, Ingrid. *Cancer Salves, A Botanical Approach to Treatment*. Publisher: Seventh Ray Press; 1999. ISBN-13: 978-1556432705

Pierce, Tanya Harte. *Outsmart Your Cancer: Alternative Non-Toxic Treatments That Work*. Publisher: Thoughtworks Publishing; 2nd edition; August 1, 2009. ISBN-13: 978-0972886789

Reilly, Harold J., and Ruth Hagy Brod. *The Edgar Cayce Handbook For Health Through Drugless Therapy*. Publisher: A.R.E. Press; September 2008. ISBN-13: 978-0876042151

Wigmore, Ann. *The Wheatgrass Book: How to Grow and Use Wheatgrass to Maximize Your Health and Vitality*. Publisher: Avery Trade; October 1, 1985. ISBN-13: 978-0895292346

Clinic Information

THE BIO-MEDICAL CENTER

Mailing Address:
P. O. Box 433654
San Ysidro, California 92143

U.S. Phone Lines:
(619) 704 8442
(619) 407 7858

Mexico Phone lines:
011 52 (664) 684 9011
011 52 (664) 684 9744, fax

Website:
None as of this writing.

Email:
Bio-Medicalcenter@prodigy.net.mx
biomedleola@gmail.com

Hours:
Monday through Friday
8:00 a.m. to 4:00 p.m., Pacific Standard Time

Newsletters, books, and videos showing the patient experience are available from the clinic.

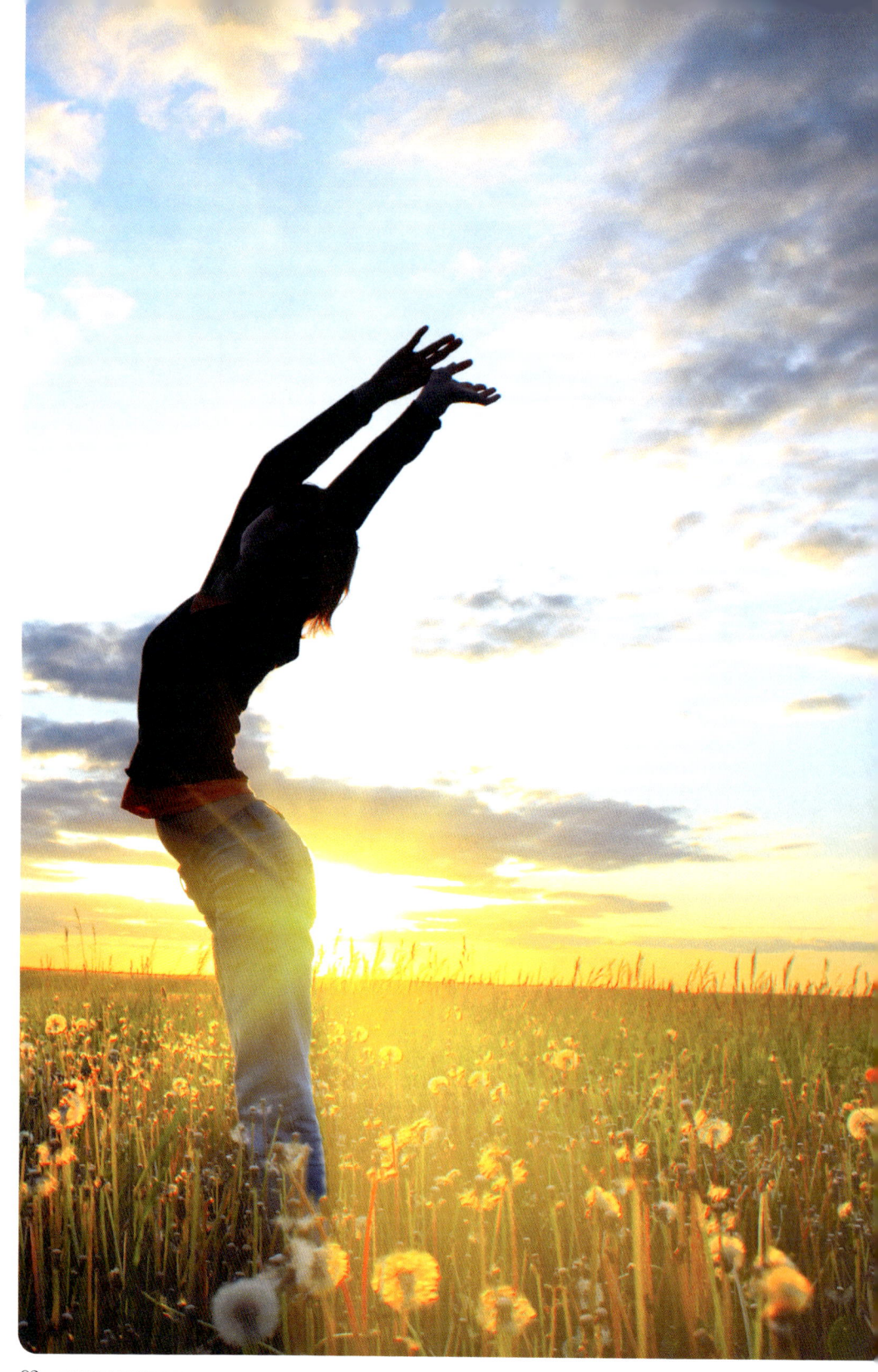

Index

A

Abrahams Osculator (Abrams' Oscillator), 22
Abrams, Albert, 22
alcohol tinctures, 14
alkaloid poisons, 23
aloe-emodin, 31, 33
American bittersweet *(Celastrus scandens)*, 75
American Cancer Society
    campaign against Hoxsey clinic, 5-6
    on cancer cure rates, 1
    1958 political campaign, 5-6
    public image of, 5-6
American mandrake, 75
American Medical Association, 5-6
American Society of Microbiology, 23
America's war on cancer, 1
anticancer herbal tea, 20
Arctium lappa. See burdock; dandelion root *(Arctium lappa)*
Artemisinin, 53
Association for Research and Enlightenment (A.R.E.), 7, 39-40, 64, 78
Ausubel, Kenny, 5-6

B

Back to Eden (Kloss), 15, 17
Baer, Susan S., 40
balm of gilead, 19
balsam of tolu, 26
barberry *(Berberis vulgaris)*, **32**
    Cayce's use of, 31
    in dry herbal capsules, 77
berberine, 31
Berberis vulgaris. See barberry
Bio-Medical Center, **3**.
    See also case studies
    clinic information, 81
    cost of treatment at, 13, 42
    description of, **3-4**
    dietary guidelines, 19

Bio-Medical Center, *continued*
    The Experience (video), 52
    herbal capsule ingredient, 77
    Hoxey therapy at, 3-4
    Roger Bloom's experience at, 2-4
    use of *Cascara sagrada,* 33
"black tonic," 53
blessed thistle, 76
blood purification, 19
bloodroot, 12, 59-60
blood toxicity, 35
Boik, John, 31
Bond, Edgar, 13
Bosnan, Mirand, 58-59
Bowers, Benjamin F., 13
Bowie, R.C., 13
breast cancer. *See also* cancer
    case study on, 42-44, 56-61, 63-67
    surgery suggested (case study), 46-51
    use of stillingia for, 31
Brinker, Francis, 17
Brown, Tom Jr., 10
buchu leaves
    for mercury and nightshade poisoning, 26
    for nerve damage, 19
buckthorn *(Rhamnus cathartica)*, **11**, 31, **32**
burdock *(Arctium lappa)*, **21**
    in anti-cancer remedy, 76
    in Caisse's tea, 8
    Cayce/Hoxsey formula, 74
    in dry herbal capsules, 77
    for energy medicine, 20-22
    in essiac tea, 76
    plant preparation, 71
    for treating blood toxicity, 35
    for treating hallucinations, 35
    for treating nerve impairment, 35
    for treating throat cancer, 20-22
Burkhart, Lona, 58-61

C

Caisse, Renee, 8, 20.
    See also herbal teas

Calborn, Cherie, 65
Calborn, John, 65
calisaya bark *(Cinchona calisaya)*, 26, 74
cancer. *See also* breast cancer; case studies; herbal formulas
    alternative therapies, physicians knowledge of, 5-6
    America's war on, 1
    breast (case study), 42-44, 56-61
    of the breast, 31
    Cayce's therapy modalities for, 7-8
    cure rates for, 2
    Hodgkins Lymphoma (case study), 51-54
    iodide potassium for, 20-22
    necrosis of cells, 11
    pancreatic (case study), 58-61
    simple syrup, for throat cancer, 22
    thyroid, 34
    1971 "war" on, 1
Cancer, Its Causes, Symptoms, and Treatment (Jones), 23-25
Cancer and Natural Medicine (Boik), 31
Cancer Control Society, 78
Cancer Industry, The (Moss), 6
Cancer Medicine From Nature (Bloom), 51, 65
Caputi, Linda, 40-41, 46-51
Caputi, Socheata, 46-51
Cascara sagrada (Rhamnus purshiana), **32**
    in anti-cancer remedy, 76
    in dry herbal capsules, 77
    uses for, 33
cascarosides, 33
case studies
    breast cancer, 42-44, 56-61, 63-67
    breast cancer, surgery suggested, 46-51
    Hodgkins lymphoma, 51-54
    pancreatic cancer, 58--61, 61-63
    prostate cancer, 44-45
    uterine cancer, 40-41
Cayce, Edgar, **7**
    approaches to cancer treatment, 7-8
    and the A.R.E., 7

Cayce, Edgar, *continued*
    Cayce/Hoxsey formula, 74
    formulae, 73-76
    praise of skepticism, 36
    tinctures and infusions, 14
chaparral leaves, 76-77
chelerythine, 28
cherry bark. *See* wild cherry bark
Chips, Allen S., 51-54
Christopher, John R., 76
common plantain *(Plantago major)*, 72
Complete Cancer Cleanse (Calborn, Calborn, Mahaffey), 65
compound syrup phytolacca, 75
compound syrup scrophularia, 75
COX-2 inhibitors, 28

D

dandelion root *(Arctium lappa)*, 71, 75
dental hygiene, 28
detoxification, nutritional caution during, 19
Dicumarol, 11
dietary guidelines
    for eliminating poisons from the body, 26
    during treatment, 19
drugs, manufacturing of, 10
Duke, James, 10
    on the Hoxsey formula, 27
    on lignans, 20
    on prickly ash, 28
    uses for licorice, 33

E

Eclectic Medicine International, 79
elder
    berries, **4**
    flower, for mercury and nightshade poisoning, 26
    flower, for treating nerve damage, 19
energy medicine, 20-22
Epilepsy-Jody's Journey (Caputi), 46
equilibrium, 33

essence of tolu, for intestinal conditions, 18
essiac tea (Caisse), 76
Experience, The (video), 52

F

Federal Drug Administration, 6
figwort *(Scrophularia nodosa)*, 75
Fishbein, Morris, 5
Fitzgerald fact-finding report, 6

G

gentian *(Gentiana lutea)*, 75
Gerson, Max, 78
Gerson Institute, 78
glycerin tinctures, 14
Glycyrrhiza glabra. See licorice
glycyrrhizic acid, 33
goldenseal *(Hydrastus canadensis)*, 72, 74
grain alcohol, 26
guaiacum wood, 75

H

hallucinations, 34
Hartwell, Jonathan
   Plants Used Against Cancer, 27-28
   use of red clover, 17
   on the use of stillingia, 31
   uses of licorice, 33
   on uses of licorice, 33
Henderson, Bill, 78
herbal formulas. *See also* Hoxsey's herbal formula; specific herbs; specific physical conditions
   anti-cancer remedy (Christopher), 76
   Bio-Medical Center dry herbal capsules, 77
   Hoxsey's, ingredients in, 12
   for intestinal conditions, 18
   for nerve damage, 19
   for throat cancer, 20-22
   tinctures and infusions used in making, 14

herbal teas
   Caisses' anticancer, 20
   Caisse's essiac tea, 76
   Winters', 76
Herbs Against Cancer (Moss), 25
HIV virus, 23
Hodgkins lymphoma, 51-54
Hoxsey, Harry
   biographical information on, 4-6
   court fights, during McCarthyism era, 6
   on Dicumarol, 11
   explanation of his formula, 11
   on external formulas, 10-11
   herbal formula ingredients, 12
   on herbal formulas, 10-11
   on potassium iodide, 11
Hoxsey clinic, Dallas, Texas, 4
Hoxsey's herbal formula. *See also* herbal formulas; specific physical conditions
   herbal formula, 74
   ingredients in, 42
   male hormone blocking drugs and, 45
   modern limitations of, 36
   physicians report on, 12-13
   suggested additions to, 12, 42
   used in veterinary medicine, 34
   use of alcohol in, 14
Hydrastus canadensis. See goldenseal

I

Indian mud, 59-60
Indian rhubarb, 76
infusions, 14
International Journal of Oncology, 53
intestinal conditions, 18
intraductal carcinoma, 42
inulin, 20
iodide potassium, for throat cancer, 20-22
isoflavones, in soy, 17

J

JAMA. *See* American Medical Association
Jason Winters Story, The (Sattilaro), 8

Jones, Eli, 20, 23-25, 72
    formulas from, 75
    stillingia for cancer, 31
juniper berries *(Juniperus communis)*, 75

K

kaempferol, 31
Kalm, Hans, 13
kelp, 76
Killing Your Cancer Without Killing Yourself (Chips), 51
Kincaid, Marion, 63-67
Kloss, Jethro, 15, 17

L

lacteal ducts, 28
licorice *(Glycyrrhiza glabra)*, **12, 32**
    in anti-cancer remedy, 76
    COX-2 components of, 33
    in dry herbal capsules, 77
    uses for, 33
lignans, 20
Linus Pauling Institute, 79
Loffler, E. E., 13
Lymphoma RX, 53

M

Mahaffey, Michael, 65
Main, Carol, 61-63
male hormone blocking drugs, 45
mandrake root *(Sassafras albidum)*, **74**
    for mercury and nightshade poisoning, 26
    for nerve damage, 19
McCarthyism in America, 6
McGarey, Bill, 64
McMakin, Carolyn, 78
mercury poisoning, 25-26
milkweed plant, 26
Moss, Ralph, 6, 25, 78
Mountain Rose Herbs, 79
Mueller, H. B., 13
Myrna (case study), 56-61

N

Naiman, Ingrid, 72, 79
National Cancer Institute, 27
National Center for Complementary and Alternative Medicine, 1, 17
Nelson, Mildred
    concern for patients, 61-63
    director, Bio-Medical Center, 6
    and the Hoxsey formulas, 10
nerve damage, 19, 35
nitidine, 28

O

Office of Alternative Medicine. *See* National Center for Complementary and Alternative Medicine
Office of Technology Assessment (OTA), 20, 25
oil of sassafras
    for intestinal conditions, 18
    sassafras tree, **37**
Options, the Alternative Cancer Therapy Book (Walters), 8
Oregon grape root *(Mahonia aquifolium)*, 76, **77**
Oregon State University, 79
OTA. *See* Office of Technology Assessment
Outsmart Your Cancer (Pierce, Tanya), 45

P

Palmer, Willard G., 13
pancreatic cancer, 58--61, 61-63
Parke, Davis and Co., 18
pau d'arco, 77
Pauling, Linus, 79
peach bark *(Prunus persica)*, 76
pelvic nerve distress, 34
Penobscot Indians, 25
Peterson Field Guides, 15
petroleum jelly, 75
phytoestrogen genistein, 17
phytolacca, compound syrup, 75
Phytolacca americana. See poke

Phytolacca folium, 75
Pierce, Tanya, 45, 79
pine *(Pinus)*, 72
plaintain, common *(Plantago major)*, 72, **73**
Plantago major. See common plantain
plantain leaves, 26
plant identification, sources for, 15
Plants Used Against Cancer (Hartwell), 27
poke *(Phytolacca americana)*, **24-25, 27**
    alkaloid poisons in, 23
    in anti-cancer remedy, 76
    anti-viral protein in, 23
    Cayce/Hoxsey formula, 74
    in compound syrup phytolacca, 75
    in compound syrup scrophularia, 75
    for intestinal conditions, 18
    for mercury and nightshade poisoning, 26
    for mercury poisoning, 25-26
    for nightshade poisoning, 25-26
    plant preparation, 71-72
    preparation of, 23
    in skin cancer ointment, 75
    for throat cancer, 20-22
    for treating hallucinations, 35
polysacharides, 20
potassium iodide, **34**
    "black tonic," 53
    in the Cayce/Hosxey herbal formula, 74
    common uses of, 34
    in the Hoxsey formula, 11
    for treating blood toxicity, 35
    for treating nerve impairment, 35
    uses for, 34
prebiotic inulin, 20
prickly ash *(Zanthoxylum americanum)*, **29**
    in anti-cancer remedy, 76
    Cayce/Hoxsey formula, 74
    in compound syrup scrophularia, 75
    for dental hygeine, 28
    in dry herbal capsules, 77
    for nerve damage, 19
prostate cancer (case study), 44-45
Prunus serotina. See wild cherry bark

Q

queen's delight. *See* stillingia

R

Rappahannock Indians, 25
Recalled By Life (Sattilaro), 8
red clover *(Trifolium pratense)*, **16, 18**
    in anti-cancer remedy, 76
    Cayce/Hoxsey formula, 74
    in dry herbal capsules, 77
    in essiac tea, 76
    for intestinal conditions, 18
    N.C.I research on, 17
    for nerve damage, 19
    plant preparation, 71
    in Winters' tea, 8
Rhamnus cathartica. See buckthorn
Rhamnus purshiana. See Cascara sagrada
rhubarb, 77
Ridge Runner Trading Company, 79
Rowen, Robert J., 53
Rumex crispus. See yellow dock root

S

sarsaparilla *(Smilax officinalis)*
    in anti-cancer remedy, 76
    Cayce/Hoxsey formula, 74
    in dry herbal capsules, 77
    for mercury and nightshade poisoning, 26
sassafras. See oil of sassafras
sassafras tree, **37**
Sattilaro, Anthony, 8
Schweitzer, Albert, 78
scrophularia, compound syrup, 75
sheep sorrel, 76
Shufer, Vickie, 10
Sikes, Barbara F., 42-44
Similax officinalis. See sarsaparilla
simple syrup, for throat cancer, 22
slippery elm, 76
Smilax officinalis. See sarsaparilla
smoking, 5

Spring Wind Herbs, 53
Starwest Botanicals, 79
stillingia *(Stillingia sylvatica)*, **30**
    in anti-cancer remedy, 76
    Cayce/Hoxsey formula, 74
    for the circulatory system, 31
    for digestion, 31
    for internal cancer, 31
    for intestinal conditions, 18
    for liver functions, 31
    for throat cancer, 20-22
    for treating blooc toxicity, 35
    for treating hallucinations, 35
    for treating nerve impairment, 35
Stillingia sylvatica. *See* stillingia
Strack, Karl, 44-45
Streptococci bacilli, 28
Swank, Roy, 42
sweet wormword, 53
syphilis, 34
syrup phytolacca, 75
Syrup Trifolium Compound (Parke, Davis, and Co.), 18

T

tamoxifen, 17, 56
taxol, 53
teas. *See* herbal teas
The Cancer Industry (Moss), 6
The Complete Cancer Cleanse (Calborn and Calborn), 65
The Experience (video), 52, 63
The Jason Winters Story (Sattilaro), 8
thistle flower, **61**
throat cancer. *See* cancer
Thurston, Frederick H., 13
thyroid cancer, 34
Timbs, A. C., 13
tinctures and infusions, 14
tolu, essence of. *See* essence of tolu
toothache bark. *See* prickly ash
trichloro-acetic acid, 12
Trifolium pratense. *See* red clover
turkey corn root, 75
turmeric, 77

U

uterine cancer (case study), 40-41

V

Venture Inward Magazine, 51
veterinary medicine, 34

W

Walters, Richard, 8
Ward, Patricia Spain
    Hoxsey treatment study, 31
    on pokeweed, 25
    research on burdock, 20
watercress, 76
websites
    cancer salves, 72
    Carol Main, 63
    distillation procedure (Jones), 75
    herbal resources, 79
    resources, 78-79
wheat grass, in Wigmore's juice, 8
When Healing Becomes a Crime (Ausubel), 5
Wigmore, Ann, 8, 78
wild cherry bark
    fruit and leaves, **9**
    for mercury and nightshade poisoning, 26
    for nerve damage, 19
    for throat cancer, 20-22
    for treating blood toxicity, 35
    for treating nerve impairment, 35
wild cherry bark *(Prunus serotina)*, 74
Winters, Jason, 8, 17, 76.
    See also herbal teas
Winters' tea, 20

Y

Yeats, Roy O., 13
yellow dock root *(Rumex crispus)*
    Cayce/Hoxsey formula, 74
    in compound syrup scrophularia, 75
    for intestinal conditions, 18

yellow dock root, *continued*
    for nerve damage, 19
    plant preparation, 71
    for throat cancer, 20-22
    for treating blood toxicity, 35
    for treating hallucinations, 35
    for treating nerve impairment, 35
yew needles, 41, 53
yew tablets, 56-57

Z

Zanthoxylum americanum.
    See prickly ash

Notes

Notes

Notes

Made in the USA
Charleston, SC
30 October 2012